T0382885

The Dignity of Labour?

Originally published in 1979, this study looks at the experience of child-bearing from three viewpoints: first and foremost from that of the child-bearing women; but in addition it considers the views and experiences of midwives and consultant obstetricians.

It examines the proportion of induced labours and questions who is induced, when, where and why and how. Comparisons are then made between induced and non-induced labours of mothers' experiences of labour and delivery and then of the babies conditions and the early relationships between the mothers and babies. Women's views of their experiences, their attitudes to the information they were given, and their choice for treatment at further pregnancies are then examined.

In the final chapter induction policies and practices are reviewed in the light of women's reactions to their experiences. The implications of the findings are discussed in relation to other innovatory and interventionist procedures and in the context of the women's movement.

The Dignity of Labour?

A Study of Childbearing and Induction

Ann Cartwright

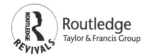

Routledge
Taylor & Francis Group

First published in 1979
by Tavistock Publications Ltd

This edition first published in 2024 by Routledge
4 Park Square, Milton Park, Abingdon, Oxon, OX14 4RN

and by Routledge
605 Third Avenue, New York, NY 10017

Routledge is an imprint of the Taylor & Francis Group, an informa business

© 1979 Ann Cartwright

All rights reserved. No part of this book may be reprinted or reproduced or utilised in any form or by any electronic, mechanical, or other means, now known or hereafter invented, including photocopying and recording, or in any information storage or retrieval system, without permission in writing from the publishers.

Publisher's Note
The publisher has gone to great lengths to ensure the quality of this reprint but points out that some imperfections in the original copies may be apparent.

Disclaimer
The publisher has made every effort to trace copyright holders and welcomes correspondence from those they have been unable to contact.

A Library of Congress record exists under ISBN: 0422766909

ISBN: 978-1-032-71903-0 (hbk)
ISBN: 978-1-032-71909-2 (ebk)
ISBN: 978-1-032-71910-8 (pbk)

Book DOI 10.4324/9781032719092

Ann Cartwright

Institute for Social Studies
in Medical Care

The Dignity of
Labour?

A Study of Childbearing
and Induction

TAVISTOCK PUBLICATIONS

First published in 1979
by Tavistock Publications Limited
11 New Fetter Lane, London EC 4P 4EE
© *Ann Cartwright 1979*
Printed in Great Britain
at the University Press, Cambridge

ISBN 0 422 76690 9

Contents

Copies of the questionnaire used in this study can be obtained from the Institute for Social Studies in Medical Care, 14 South Hill Park, London NW3 2SB.

Acknowledgements

I am very grateful to the many people who helped and contributed to this study:

The mothers, doctors, and midwives who answered our many questions – and particular thanks are due to the women who had had a still birth and went over their experiences for our benefit.

The interviewers who persuaded them to do this, particularly Hilary Gellman, Flo Green, Margery Thorne, and the late Muriel Toney, who supervised.

Maureen O'Brien, who helped at all stages.

Other colleagues at the Institute for Social Studies in Medical Care, and most notably Janet Ball who typed innumerable documents and sent out postal questionnaires and reminders, and Christopher Smith who has checked much of this report and helped with the appendices.

Ian Hutchinson and his colleagues at the Office of Population Censuses and Surveys who selected the sample of births, Mr Nickless at the DHSS who gave us a list of consultants in obstetrics and gynaecology, and the nursing officers at the hospitals who sent us lists of the midwives who were working there.

The Royal Colleges of General Practitioners, of Midwives, and of Obstetricians and Gynaecologists, which all expressed support for the study.

The Institute's Advisory Committee, who supported and advised at various stages: Abe Adelstein, Tony Alment, Val Beral, Vera

viii   Acknowledgements

Carstairs, May Clarke, Spence Galbraith, Geoffrey Hawthorn, Austin Heady (Chairperson), Margot Jefferys, Joyce Leeson, John McEwan, David Morrell, Martin Richards.

The DHSS, which supported the study, and particularly Doreen Rothman, Arthur Forsdick, Marguerite Smith, and Audrey King.

The coders, including Margaret Hall, Ming Moseley-Williams, Richard Mond, and Pete Bastick.

The machine operators and punchers, Joan Deane, Suzan Gomez, Dorothy Hills, Louise Holland, Ann Pentol, and Alison Venning.

Iain Chalmers, who commented at many stages and also helped with the classification of causes of still birth.

Alwyn Smith and his colleagues at the Department of Community Medicine at Manchester, who gave hospitality and support.

People who helped in various other ways including Eva Alberman, Richard Beard, Gwen Cartwright, Audrey Chamberlain, Geoffrey Chamberlain, Vivien Hillier, Peter Huntingford, Jean Robinson, Wyn Tucker, Michael Wadsworth, and Jo Weatherall.

1 Introduction

In recent years obstetric care has been increasingly interventionist and more and more babies have been born in hospital. In 1959, 64 per cent of the births in England and Wales were in hospital. Ten years later this proportion had increased to 84 per cent, and by 1974 the proportion in England was 96 per cent (DHSS 1977a: 142).[1] Between 1958 and 1970 the proportion of births delivered by Caesarean section rose from 2.7 per cent to 4.5 per cent, and the proportion for which forceps were used from 4.7 per cent to 7.9 per cent (Chamberlain *et al.* 1975: 29). But it is the rise in induction from an estimated 15 per cent in 1965 to around 41 per cent in 1974 (DHSS 1976: 60; DHSS 1977b: 77) that has attracted the most publicity and concern. The benefits and disadvantages of induction on such a widespread scale are being debated and questioned in the lay and in the medical press and by social scientists. Basically, three possible reasons for the increased use of induction are put forward.

Possible reasons for the increase in inductions

First, there is the argument put forward by some obstetricians that it has reduced perinatal mortality, led to shorter labours, and babies generally being born in a healthier state (Tipton and Lewis 1975). Dugald Baird in 1960 claimed that 'our investigations suggested that there is much to be said for induction of labour to avoid the risk of

[1] References are given in full at the end of the book.

placental insufficiency which increases with prolonged pregnancy' and that this policy had led to a big decrease in unexplained and asphyxial deaths, and those from birth trauma. These observations encouraged other obstetricians to try to reduce perinatal mortality rates in their areas by increasing the proportion of inductions. And during this time the perinatal mortality rate fell, from 34.1 in England and Wales in 1959 to 23.4 in 1969 (DHSS 1977a: 14), and in England in 1975 it was below 20 for the first time. A leader in the *British Medical Journal* in 1976 affirmed: 'Obstetrics is one of the few areas of medicine in which in the last decade technological innovation has not only been rapid but has proved to be effective'. But, of course, changes in age, parity, nutrition, height, and other social characteristics of mothers contribute to changes in perinatal mortality rate. Not all obstetricians accept the argument that a high level of induction has contributed to the reduction in perinatal mortality, and there is an increasing amount of evidence to shed doubt on this assumption.

The second explanation for the increase in inductions comes largely from social scientists. Martin Richards argues that it 'reflects a tradition in obstetrics that favours interventionist procedures which involve close control over patients and appear to be "scientific"' (1975). He points to the lack of appropriate quality control in obstetrics and suggests that professional dominance has allowed this irrational practice to persist. Some paediatricians have taken a similar line. Dunn (1976), discussing current obstetric practice, quotes the Director-General of the World Health Organization (Mahler 1975) as saying: 'It is frightening, but expected, that when a specialised group is formed to perform certain actions, it is evaluated and continues to be supported because of the *number* of such actions which it does, rather than by whether a problem is solved'. Dunn, commenting on the frequency of interventions, feels that they have almost become part of the ritual of modern delivery and wonders whether some obstetricians have become intoxicated by their new technology.

Third, inductions may have increased for reasons of convenience. This aspect has been emphasized by the lay press and by patients' representatives. A review in the *Sunday Times* stated: 'Technology is now being used in some hospitals to induce births routinely, not primarily for the baby's safety or the safety of the mother, but in order to create a production line system where women have their babies by clockwork during daylight hours' (Gillie and Gillie 1974). And an article on mothers' reactions to induction was headlined *Battery Hen*

Mothers and Conveyor Belt Babies (Robinson 1974). Certainly some obstetricians regarded a high induction rate as a reasonable policy in a situation of staff shortages, and in some hospitals two-thirds of the births were induced (Walker, Martin, and Higginbottom 1972).

Studies of induction

Most of the studies of induction have been concerned with the possible effects on the life and health of the mothers and babies. In 1968, Anderson, Turnbull, and Baird reviewed the influence of induction of labour on Caesarean section rate, duration of labour, and perinatal mortality among primigravidae in Aberdeen between 1938 and 1966. They concluded that 'the liberal use of induction of labour has undoubtedly helped to lower the perinatal mortality rate in Aberdeen'. In support, they quoted 'the results of the Perinatal Mortality Survey (1968) which shows that in 1958 in the United Kingdom the incidence of prolonged pregnancy and of perinatal deaths associated with it in primigravidae was considerably higher than in Aberdeen'. They ended: 'Today young women are taller and healthier than their mothers. They marry and have their first child at an earlier age. These changes in themselves must lower the incidence of difficult labour from disproportion and from dysfunction and decrease the need for oxytocin infusion and Caesarean section in labour. The beneficial effects of the improved health and physique of mothers will also show itself in increased reproductive efficiency in general. This is already one of the factors in the rapid fall in perinatal mortality in the United Kingdom since 1958'. Baird and Thomson, reviewing the Aberdeen findings, concluded: 'Perinatal deaths occurring after term are characterised by post-mortem signs of asphyxia or mechanical stress, and death rates from such causes can be considerably reduced by a selective policy of induction of labour and avoidance of prolonged and difficult labour' (1969).

More recently, a large series of births in Cardiff has been analysed. Chalmers *et al.* (1976), reviewing trends from 1965 to 1973, report an increase in inductions from 7.5 per cent to 26.5 per cent but no significant change in the perinatal mortality rate.

Another centre with data about all deliveries in a geographical area is Oxford. Here the induction rate increased from 22.2 per cent in 1965 to 35.7 per cent in 1972 (Fedrick and Yudkin 1976). In Oxford, unlike Cardiff, the perinatal mortality rate fell from 20 per 1,000 in 1965 to 16

4 The Dignity of Labour?

per 1,000 in 1972. Fedrick and Yudkin conclude that this fall 'can be explained partly by a reduction in the proportion of high-risk elderly women and those of high parity and low social class, but changes in obstetric practice may also have caused an overall reduction, especially in still births' (1976).

McNay *et al.*, analysing births at Glasgow Royal Maternity Hospital during the ten years 1966 to 1975, report that the proportion of induced births had increased from 16.3 per cent to 35.6 per cent. 'During the same period perinatal mortality fell from 33 to 22 per 1,000 . . . The reduction in the number of deaths of unknown causes in mature fetuses was achieved by preventing deaths occurring after 40 weeks and was recorded in all age and parity groups. The results suggested that increased use of induction of labour has contributed to the improved perinatal mortality rate' (1977). Their conclusion has been criticized on the grounds that only hospital deliveries were included in their study (Chalmers, Newcombe, and Campbell 1977) and it has been pointed out that 'the increase in induction seems to have been associated in Glasgow with an interruption in the generally downward trend [in perinatal mortality rates] in the earlier years' (Leeson and Smith 1977).

All the studies discussed so far depend on trends over time, and there is the problem that other factors may be changing as well as obstetric practice on induction. Another study in Glasgow attempted a prospective randomized trial of elective induction (Cole, Howie, and Macnaughton 1975). It covered 'a hundred and eleven obstetrically normal pregnant women who had elective induction of labour performed between 39 and 40 weeks' and '117 controls who were managed expectantly until 41 weeks'. In the event, 46 per cent of the controls were induced (19 per cent before forty-one weeks because of an obstetric complication and 27 per cent because their pregnancies were prolonged beyond forty-one weeks). In any event their numbers were too small to give any useful data on perinatal mortality. In another prospective study of 1,000 consecutive primigravidae, labour was induced on ninety-five occasions. None of sixteen perinatal deaths and none of four cases of suspected brain damage occurred after prolonged pregnancy or pre-eclampsia. It is concluded that 'a low incidence of induction is compatible with good results' (O'Driscoll, Carroll, and Coughlan 1975). Again the study covered a relatively small number of births.

A more fruitful source of information has been the Cardiff Births

Survey with a comparison of two obstetric teams with widely differing practices and attitudes on induction. Between them the teams supervised the delivery of nearly 10,000 babies in the study period. One team did almost twice as many inductions as the other, proportionately, but 'after controlling for differences in the attributes of the two groups of patients treated, it was not possible to show any striking advantage or disadvantage of the more active approach' (Chalmers, Lawson, and Turnbull 1976).

At the same time as the clinical advantages of an enthusiastic interventionist obstetric policy are being challenged, the potentially deleterious effects on the experience of labour for the mother are increasingly discussed.

There have been several reports in the press along the lines that 'the human side of childbirth is often forgotten in the busy hospital routine which can reduce an otherwise sane woman to an emotional wreck' (Gillie and Gillie 1974). In an analysis of letters in response to a programme on *Woman's Hour*, Robinson (1974) reported that 75 per cent of women who had been induced were against it. Kitzinger (1975) analysed 614 reports of pharmacologically induced labours and 224 of non-induced ones. All the mothers had attended National Childbirth Trust ante-natal classes. She found that, for many women, induction of labour was associated with extremely painful labour, exclusion of the husband from delivery, separation of mother and neonate, and 'distress, which was increased by failure to give adequate information, encouragement, and comfort' (1975).

But studies based on women writing to the BBC or women attending National Childbirth Trust classes are almost certainly biased towards the articulate and the middle classes. A prospective study of 200 patients at a single hospital found that 45 per cent of the induced patients reported that labour had been more painful than expected, compared with 33 per cent of the spontaneous group–although patients generally expected induced labour to be more painful. But the doctors who carried out this study concluded that 'a high degree of patient acceptability can be obtained by careful explanation of induction of labour' (Lewis, Rana, and Crook 1975).

But there are no surveys or systematic assessments of women's views on a wide and representative scale. This study tries to fill that gap. In addition it provides data, not elsewhere available, about who is induced and when, why, and how these inductions are carried out.

6 The Dignity of Labour?

This study

This study looks at the experience of childbearing from three viewpoints: first and foremost from that of the childbearing women; but in addition it considers the views and experiences of midwives and consultant obstetricians.

The survey of mothers was carried out in twenty-four randomly selected areas of England and Wales.[2] In each area fifty legitimate births registered during July 1975 and fifty registered during August were selected at random by the Office of Population Censuses and Surveys. Out of this sample of 2,400, 91 per cent were successfully interviewed. In addition, a sample of 240 legitimate still births, ten in each of the twenty-four areas, was taken. These were spread over a rather wider geographical area in order to build up sufficient numbers. The response rate among the women who had had a still birth was somewhat lower, 82 per cent.[3] The reasons for failure are shown in *Table 1.*

Table 1 The response of mothers

	Live births		Still births	
	Number	%	*Number*	%
Successfully interviewed	2182	90.9	196	81.7
Refused	99	4.1	22	9.2
Not contacted	21	0.9	7	2.9
Moved – not known where to	62	2.6	5	2.1
Moved out of country	35	1.5	7	2.9
Mother died	1	—	—	—
Not eligible*	—	—	3	1.2
Total	2400	100.0	240	100.0

* Three of the selected still births were illegitimate.

Those who had had a still birth were both more elusive and more likely to refuse than those with a live born baby.

Of those interviewed, 7 per cent had moved within the study area and 1 per cent outside it. An interpreter was used for 3 per cent of the interviews. The interval between the birth and the interview is shown in *Table 2.*

[2] The way this was done is described in *Appendix I*, where further details of the sample are also given.

[3] For a discussion of statistical significance see *Appendix II*.

Table 2 Interval between birth and interview

	Live births	Still births
	%	%
Less than 3 months	9	10
3 months < 4 months	56	59
4 months < 5 months	30	26
5 months < 6 months	4	5
6 months or longer	1	—
*Number of births (= 100%)**	2175	196

* Small numbers for whom inadequate information was obtained have been omitted in this and in subsequent tables.

Almost two-thirds of the mothers were seen within four months of the birth, and 95 per cent within five months. Half of the interviews lasted between an hour and a half and two hours, a fifth took less than an hour and a half, and a third more than two hours. A structured questionnaire was used.[4] It started by asking for information about all of their pregnancies and then went in detail through the pregnancy leading to the study baby: ante-natal care, arrangements for the birth, symptoms, and anxieties. This was followed by questions about labour, delivery, post-natal care, and attitudes to possible future pregnancies and maternity care.

To get a picture of the views and experiences of people responsible for obstetric practices and policies, letters and questionnaires were sent to all of the 679 people listed as consultants in obstetrics or gynaecology by the Department of Health and Social Security. Twelve replied to say they did not do any obstetrics, five had died, thirteen had retired. Among the remaining 649, 379 or 58 per cent returned a completed questionnaire, 11 per cent wrote refusing to do so, 2 per cent were returned because the consultant was no long at the address or was temporarily working abroad, and 29 per cent failed to reply after one written and one telephone reminder. The response rate was 65 per cent among those aged under forty and 51 per cent among those aged sixty or more. It was higher (73 per cent) among those with full-time university appointments than among those with NHS ones (57 per cent). It did not vary with the sex of the consultant, and it was similar

[4] Copies of the questionnaire can be obtained from the Institute for Social Studies in Medical Care, 14 South Hill Park, London NW3 2SB. A charge will be made for photocopying when supplies run out.

for those born inside Great Britain and for those born elsewhere. Unfortunately, no other data are available about the consultants who did not respond.

The sample of midwives was obtained by writing to area nursing officers responsible for all the hospitals and nursing homes at which five or more of the initial sample of live births took place, and asking them for a list of midwives currently working in the hospital. The lists were then sampled in proportion to the number of sample births at the hospital, and to give a total of twenty midwives in each of the twenty-four areas, i.e. a total of 480 in all. Interviews were obtained with 388, that is, 81 per cent. The main reason for failure was the refusal or neglect of the area nursing officers to let us have a list. This accounted for 13 per cent of the failures. Three per cent of the midwives approached refused, and there were a variety of reasons among the other 3 per cent.

Finally an attempt was made to compare some of the medical information obtained from mothers with data available from medical records. A random one in ten of those interviewed who had had a live birth and all those who had had a still birth were asked if they were willing for us to get in touch with their doctor or the hospital to get some medical information about their pregnancy and confinement. Seven per cent of those who had had a live birth and 11 per cent of those with a still birth did not agree, so no medical information was sought for them. In addition, no attempt was made to collect medical data about those who had had a home birth. Among those for whom medical information was sought, it was obtained for 131 out of the 191 live births, 69 per cent, and 109 out of the 168 still births, 65 per cent – not a significant difference. The person who completed the form for the live births was most often a consultant (56 per cent) or general practitioner (18 per cent). Nine per cent were filled in by a registrar, 5 per cent by a house officer, 7 per cent by a midwife, and 5 per cent by a clerk. For convenience they are all referred to as doctors. Forms were no more or less likely to be completed for women who reported an induction than for those whose labour started spontaneously.

The questions to be answered

Data are available from other sources about the proportion of labours that are induced, but not about who is induced and when, where, why, and how. These questions are tackled first. After that comparisons are made between induced and non-induced labours of mothers' experiences of labour and delivery and then of the babies' conditions and the early relationships between the mothers and babies. Women's views of their experiences, their attitudes to the information they were given, and their choice for treatment at further pregnancies are then examined.

What are the views and experiences of obstetricians and midwives in relation to induction? These are described and compared in later chapters.

In the final chapter induction policies and practices are reviewed in the light of women's reactions to their experiences. The implications of the findings are discussed in relation to other innovatory and interventionist procedures and in the context of the women's movement.

2 What is induction? Who is induced? Why? and When?

The onset of labour may be encouraged in a number of ways. Traditionally it was done by castor oil, hot baths, and enemas (OBEs!). It can also be done surgically by artificial rupture of the membranes (ARM) or by a membrane sweep. More recently, drugs (oxytocin or prostaglandins) have been used, with or without other methods. This chapter starts with a discussion of the problems of definition and of collecting reliable information about induction.

Definition of induction

Whether a labour is induced is not always easy to define or to determine. In addition to the problem of the different methods that may be used, there is the further problem that either ARM or drugs may be given after labour has started spontaneously to facilitate or accelerate labour. If this happened it has been regarded as an 'acceleration' rather than an 'induction'. The problem then is to ascertain whether or not labour started spontaneously. After the pilot study, spontaneous labour was defined as either contractions starting or membranes rupturing spontaneously before a drip or injection was given to start labour or before membranes were ruptured artificially or there was a membrane sweep. But it was not always straightforward to apply this definition. Some problems were pains or weak contractions which might or might not have been labour starting spontaneously; a 'leak' which might or might not have been membranes rupturing spontaneously; or a drip or injection being given which might or might not have contained a drug to start labour. In the end, the interviewer's and coder's assessments of replies to a series of questions were taken. In 94 per cent of instances their assessment tallied with the mothers' responses to a direct question about whether they went into labour of their own accord or whether the doctors or nurses did anything at all to help *start* the labour. Nine mothers (less than 0.5 per cent) said labour started spontaneously when other data suggested it was induced; rather more, 3 per cent, said they were induced although other information indicated that labour started spontaneously. For the remainder, either the mother or the coder did not make an assessment.

The proportion classified as induced by this procedure and the methods used are shown in *Table 3*. This suggests that just under a quarter of the mothers had their labour induced, 2 per cent had an elective Caesarean section, and nearly three-quarters went into labour spontaneously. Two-thirds of those who were induced were given both drugs and an ARM.

Table 3 Methods of induction

	Number	%
Planned Caesarean section	48	2.2
Induced by ARM only	84	3.8
Induced by drugs only	78	3.6
Induced by both drugs and ARM	354	16.2
Induced by membrane sweep	6	0.3
Uncertain if induced	13	0.6
Labour started spontaneously	1599	73.3
Number of mothers (= 100%)	2182	100.0

(ARM only, drugs only, both, membrane sweep: }23.9)

Comparison with medical records

A comparison of the 131 live births for which information was obtained from both the mothers and doctors is given in *Table 4*.

The information tallied in 115 instances (88 per cent) and the proportion of induced births was 29 per cent[1] according to the mothers, slightly higher, 32 per cent, according to the doctors.

In six of the nine cases described by the doctors as induced and by

[1] This does not differ significantly from the 25 per cent reported for the total sample of hospital births.

12   The Dignity of Labour?

Table 4   Information about induction from mothers and doctors

Doctor reported	Mother reported			Total
	Planned Caesarean section	Induced	Labour started spontaneously	
Planned Caesarean section	4	—	—	4
Induced	—	32	9	41
Labour started spontaneously	—	6	79	85
Inadequate information	—	—	1	1
Total	4	38	89	131

the mothers as starting spontaneously, the mothers said their labour had been accelerated: 'I was given pitocin to strengthen the labour – to help things along'; 'The doctor who examined me said I'd be down for an induction but the following day I went into labour first.' In another instance the doctor recorded that labour was induced by a membrane sweep, whereas the patient said she had been given 'a fierce internal'.

One mother said by the doctor to have been induced reported that nothing had been done either to start her labour or to hurry it up, but she had been given a drip with glucose and 'something I needed in my blood in it – I'm very anaemic'. The remaining mother in this group reported no intervention except for an injection to give pain relief.

Confusion between induction and acceleration seemed to contribute to two of the six discrepancies which the doctor said were spontaneous and the mother said were induced. One mother said her labour was started by both drugs and ARM but the medical notes described her labour as being accelerated by both these methods. The other mother said her membranes were ruptured to start her labour but later the machine monitoring the baby's heart was 'dipping' so she was transferred to another hospital where she was put on a drip to accelerate it. The medical records just indicated an acceleration by oxytocin. Another mother regarded her labour as induced by drugs but the doctor who extracted the data from the medical records did not regard it as induced. This mother said:

'They put me on a drip on Wednesday from 1.30 p.m. to 10.30 p.m. that evening and then said they were going to give me two days' rest and start again on the Saturday. But the contractions started on the Thursday. They said they didn't know whether they were related to the drip or whether I started on my own.'

She also said her labour was accelerated by ARM, and this tallied with the medical record.

Another mother in this group also had an experience that seemed difficult to categorize: 'I was contracting, she said, but it wasn't proper labour so she gave me a needle to start me off properly.' However, according to the medical information her labour was neither induced nor accelerated.

The remaining two mothers in this group reported that their labour had been started by ARM: one said this had been done by the midwife at home before an emergency admission to hospital. Neither induction nor acceleration were recorded by the doctors.

The comparisons show that it is not always easy to identify the births that are induced, and confusion between acceleration and induction contributes to the problem. In some ways it might be more appropriate to identify births in which there was active management by drugs or ARM at any stage. Unfortunately, comparisons with data from medical records show many discrepancies with mothers' reports over acceleration. This can be seen from *Table 5*.

Accelerations were more often reported by mothers than recorded by doctors. Over half the labours said by the mothers to have been accelerated but not induced were recorded by the doctors as being neither accelerated nor induced. Of these twenty-two labours, half were said to have been accelerated by drugs, half by ARM alone. Over a third of the accelerations without inductions recorded by the doctors were described by the mothers as having been neither induced nor accelerated; most of them (seven out of the eight) were said to have been accelerated by ARM.

What are the possible reasons for the discrepancies? One is that accelerations may not always be recorded in the medical notes or recalled by the doctors who completed the questionnaires. Information about induction but not about acceleration is recorded for the Hospital In-Patients Enquiry. The notes about completing this form explained that surgical induction should only be ticked if sweeping or rupture of the membranes was carried out surgically in

Table 5 Information about induction and acceleration from mothers and doctors

Doctor reported	Mother reported				Total
	Planned Caesarean section	Induced	Accelerated not induced	Neither	
Planned Caesarean section	4	—	—	—	4
Induced	—	32	6	3	41
Accelerated but not induced	—	3	10	8	21
Neither accelerated nor induced	—	3	22	37*	62
Inadequate information	—	—	3	—	3
Total	4	38	41	48	131

* Includes two for which both mother and doctor reported an emergency Caesarean section.

order to initiate labour and should *not* be ticked if the membranes were ruptured *during* labour. There is no such qualification for ticking oxytocic induction. This might explain why some mothers reported acceleration by A R M or drugs when doctors recorded no acceleration or induction, and why some mothers reported acceleration by drugs when the doctors reported induction by drugs.[2] A probable reason for procedures being reported by doctors but not by mothers is that some mothers did not realize the contents or purpose of the drugs they were given or the reason for certain procedures. But there was no indication that the proportion of discrepancies was greater among first than among subsequent births.

Comparisons of procedures to either induce or accelerate are shown in *Tables 6* and *7*. *Table 6* relates to drugs and *Table 7* to artificial rupture of the membranes.

[2] Of the six labours reported by doctors as induced and by mothers as accelerated and not induced, two were said by the doctor to have been induced by drugs only (both of the mothers said they were accelerated by drugs only) and four were said to have been induced by both drugs and A R M. One of these four mothers said her labour was accelerated by drugs only, one that it was done by A R M only, and two that it was done by both.

Table 6   Information about drugs for induction or acceleration from mothers and doctors

Doctor reported drugs	Mother reported drugs		Total
	Yes	*No*	
Yes	39	6	45
No	16	63	79
Inadequate information	1	2	3
Total	56	71	127*

* The four who had planned Caesarean sections have been omitted.

Table 7   Information about ARM for induction or acceleration from mothers and doctors

Doctor reported ARM	Mother reported ARM		Total
	Yes	*No*	
Yes	34	11	45
No	24	55	79
Inadequate information	2	1	3
Total	60	67	127*

* The four who had planned Caesarean sections have been omitted.

When information was available from the two sources it tallied in 82 per cent of instances for drugs and 72 per cent for ARM. Both procedures were reported more often by mothers than by doctors.

To sum up, taking the mothers' reports of a *positive* procedure, the data from the medical records supported these in thirty-two out of thirty-eight, 84 per cent of the reports of induction; in ten out of thirty-eight, 26 per cent of the reports of acceleration without induction; in thirty-nine out of fifty-five, 71 per cent of the reports of drugs for induction or acceleration; and in thirty-four out of fifty-eight, 59 per cent of the reports of ARM for induction or acceleration.

Mothers' reports that *no* procedure was carried out tallied for seventy-nine out of eighty-eight, 90 per cent instances of no induction, thirty-seven out of forty-eight, 77 per cent instances of no induction or acceleration; sixty-three out of sixty-nine, 91 per cent of no drugs for induction or acceleration; and fifty-five out of sixty-six, 83 per cent of no A R M for induction or acceleration.

These levels seem acceptable for induction but not for acceleration or for specific interventions (drugs or A R M), so most of the comparisons that follow relate simply to 'induced' and 'non-induced' labours.

How many inductions?

Mothers reported that 24 per cent of the births were induced, and if home births are excluded the proportion is 25 per cent. Another national survey covering illegitimate as well as legitimate births in 1975 found that 27 per cent were induced (Martin 1978). Data from the Hospitals In-Patient Enquiry suggest that in 1974 the proportion was 41 per cent and that by 1975, the year of the study, it had fallen slightly to a provisional 38 per cent (D H S S 1977b: 77). There is still a substantial difference between the surveys and the H I P E data, which is probably explained by the more stringent definition in the surveys. As explained earlier, in the notes for completing the H I P E maternity form there is no indication that 'oxytocic induction' should not be ticked if oxytocin was only given after labour started. If it were given to accelerate or augment labour, the person filling in the form may have felt they ought to record this fact somewhere and this would have been the only appropriate place.

Figures available from a number of hospitals suggest that the proportion of inductions may now be declining at certain centres. In Queen Charlotte's the proportion was 31.4 per cent in 1971, 26.0 per cent in 1974. At Upton and Heatherwood hospitals it declined from 41.1 per cent in 1973 to 17.9 per cent during the first three quarters of 1975. In Cardiff the proportion fell between 1972 and 1973. (See Beard *et al.* 1976). But, as Dunn has pointed out, 'Statistics seem to be collected only in the better centres' (Beard *et al.* 1976: 23).

Data from the consultant obstetricians on this study do not suggest there had been a large drop. Early in 1976 they were asked whether more, fewer, or about the same proportion of inductions were being done 'now' compared with two years ago among the deliveries booked under their care: 73 per cent said it was about the same proportion, 20 per cent that more were being done 'now', and 7 per cent said fewer 'now'. But the level of induction they reported was roughly similar to that reported among the mothers.

When asked to estimate the proportion of births under their care that were induced, 7 per cent did not make an estimate. The distribution of the others was:

	%
60% or more	1
50% < 60%	4
40% < 50%	9
30% < 40%	23
20% < 30%	42
10% < 20%	18
5% < 10%	2
Less than 5%	1
None	–

$$100\% = 354$$

This suggests an average of around 28 per cent. This is a crude estimate based on midpoints. In addition, it gives equal weight to each consultant who replied, and, of course, consultants are responsible for different numbers of births.

So there is a puzzle. The level of induction found in this study is considerably lower than in the HIPE, but the separate estimates from mothers and obstetricians are reasonably consistent, as is the information from the two sources in our sub-sample. A more rigorous definition in this study is probably the reason for the discrepancy, but there is still the question about recent trends in the induction rate. Data from HIPE and from selected hospitals suggest this may be falling. But, if this is so, the obstetricians who responded to this study are somewhat atypical or are not fully aware of trends within their own departments.

Area and hospital variations

Turning now to the question 'Who was induced?', the first series of factors that are examined are organizational ones.

Other studies have indicated that policy over induction varies greatly (Chalmers, Lawson, and Turnbull 1976). In this study the proportions that were induced in the twenty-four study areas ranged from 6 per cent to 39 per cent. This wide variation was only marginally affected by the different proportion of home births. (The proportion of home births in the study areas varied from none to 16 per cent, but was 4 per cent in the area with the lowest proportion of inductions, and 2 per cent in the area with the highest.) Variations in size of hospital accounted for a larger part of the difference. A relatively small proportion of women giving birth in smaller hospitals with less than 100 beds were induced: 14 per cent compared with 27 per cent of those in larger hospitals. (Data about the number of beds were taken from *The Hospitals and Health Services Year Book 1975*.) If births in these small hospitals are excluded, the variation in the proportion of hospital births that were induced was from 12 per cent to 40 per cent in the study areas.

Table 8   Induction by type and size of hospital

	Proportion induced					
	Type of hospital					All hospital births
Number of beds	'Teaching'	'Non-teaching' acute	Maternity	G.P.	Other	
Under 50	9% (35)	18% (33)	20% (97)	2% (82)	*	14% (261)
50 < 100	*	17% (48)	*	*	*	14% (59)
100 < 200	22% (74)	21% (199)	27% (142)	15%**(20)	14% (29)	22% (464)
200 < 300	*	31% (119)	40% (90)	*	*	35% (209)
300 < 400	*	32% (104)	*	*	*	32% (104)
400 < 500	*	31% (241)	*	*	*	31% (241)
500 < 1000	19% (138)	24% (418)	*	*	*	23% (556)
1000 or more	37% (41)	34% (125)	*	*	*	35% (166)
All hospital births	21% (289)	27% (1287)	29% (329)	5% (105)	22% (50)	25% (2060)

Note: Figures in brackets are the numbers on which the percentages are based (= 100%).

  * No observations or inadequate numbers.
  ** This relates to one hospital with geriatric beds as well as maternity ones.

Looking at the data for individual hospitals, there were thirty-seven hospitals at which twenty or more of the study births occurred. Within these, the proportion of inductions varied from 0 per cent to 57 per cent or from 4 per cent to 57 per cent if general practitioner hospitals or maternity homes are excluded.

When the type of hospital (also taken from *The Hospitals and Health Services Year Book 1975*)[3] is considered, the proportion of inductions was

[3] The classification into 'teaching' or 'non-teaching' hospitals relates to the health districts they were in.

slightly lower at 'teaching' than at 'non-teaching' N H S hospitals, 21 per cent compared with 27 per cent. Five per cent of the births took place in general practitioner hospitals or maternity homes, and only 5 per cent of these were induced (all but one by A R M only).

The relationships between induction and type and size of hospital are shown in *Table 8*. Both size and type of hospital relate to induction independently.

The small proportion of women (less than 2 per cent) who had their babies privately rather than under the N H S were relatively likely to have an induction: 44 per cent of them did so against 24 per cent of the others.

So these institutional attributes – size of hospital, type of hospital, being a private or N H S patient, and area—were each related to induction. What about the individual characteristics of the mothers?

Age and parity

The data in relation to age and parity are shown in *Table 9*. (Parity was taken as the number of previous pregnancies ending in a live or a still birth.) The striking thing is the *lack* of variation.

If anything, a slightly higher proportion of mothers under twenty-five were induced, 27 per cent compared with 22 per cent of older

Table 9 Inductions by age and by parity

	Proportion having an elective Caesarean section	Proportion induced	Number of mothers (= 100%)
Mother's age			
Under 20	1%	24%	144
20–24	2%	28%	690
25–29	2%	21%	897
30–34	3%	28%	330
35 or more	5%	17%	104
Mother's parity			
0	2%	26%	816
1	2%	24%	853
2	3%	20%	325
3	—	24%	126
4 or more	2%	23%	47

Table 10   Inductions by age and parity

Parity	Proportion induced				
	Age of mother				
	Under 20	20–24	25–29	30–34	35+
0	29% (117)	29% (322)	22% (291)	29% (86)	
1	} 0% (26)	26% (268)	21% (414)	28% (123)	21% (24)
2		29% (80)	15% (131)	25% (88)	5% (20)
3 or more	—	20% (20)	21% (61)	31% (49)	21% (43)

Note: Figures in brackets are numbers on which percentages are based (= 100%).

mothers. This is surprising. Other data (Fedrick and Yudkin 1976) show an increasing proportion of inductions with age from 21 per cent of the under twenties to 28 per cent among those aged thirty-five or more in 1965–8, and from 27 per cent to 37 per cent in 1969–72. And earlier, before oxytocin and prostaglandins were used for induction, the induction rate reported by Baird (1960) was much higher for women aged thirty-five or more. McNay *et al.* (1977) reported an increasing induction rate with age from 16.6 per cent for those under twenty to 21.4 per cent for those aged thirty-five or more in 1966–70, but that in 1971–4, with a much higher induction rate, the variation with maternal age was no longer clear-cut. The greater precision with which fetal distress can be detected may contribute to changing patterns in the use of induction.

Fedrick and Yudkin (1976) also reported that inductions were more often prescribed for either primiparae or grand multiparae (four or more). There was some suggestion in this study, although it did not reach the level of statistical significance, that women having their first labour may be slightly more likely to be induced than others, but no evidence that induction was more common for high parity women. A three-way analysis of age, parity, and induction is given in *Table 10.*

Again, no clear-cut differences emerged, but of course individual hospitals or consultants may have definite patterns and policies.

Previous obstetric history

One possible indication for induction may be an earlier still birth because of placental insufficiency. Women who reported a previous still birth may have been marginally more likely to have an induction,

Table 11   Inductions and previous obstetric history

	Proportion having an elective Caesarean section	Proportion induced	Number of mothers (= 100%)
Still birth			
Yes	12%	30%	43
No	2%	24%	2117
Abortion			
Yes	2%	22%	58
No	2%	24%	2102
Miscarriage			
Yes	5%	25%	369
No	2%	24%	1791

but the difference, shown in *Table 11*, might easily have occurred by chance. There was, however, a difference in their Caesarean section rate.

There was no indication that a previous abortion was related to either induction or Caesarean section, but those who had had a miscarriage were more likely to have a Caesarean section though no more likely to be induced. In this connection it is relevant to note that among those for whom data were obtained from the medical records, only half of the still births or miscarriages reported by the mothers were apparently recorded in the notes.[4]

Social class

Social class[5] variations shown in *Table 12* are rather puzzling. The proportion who were induced was 21 per cent for the middle class (wives of non-manual workers) and did not vary between the three subgroups. Rather more of the working class (married to manual workers) were induced, 26 per cent, but within the working class there was a significant variation with fewest of those married to unskilled

[4] For a full comparison of data from the interviews and data from the medical records see Cartwright and Smith (in press).
[5] The index of social class was the father's occupation, as recorded on the birth certificate, classified according to the six social class groups distinguished in the Registrar General's Classification of Occupations (Office of Population Censuses and Surveys 1970). See *Appendix III* for details.

22 The Dignity of Labour?

Table 12   Inductions by social class

Social class	Proportion having an elective Caesarean section	Proportion induced	Number of mothers (= 100%)
I Professional	4%	20%	193
II Intermediate	2%	21%	367
III Skilled {Non-manual	1%	21%	239
III Skilled {Manual	2%	26%	853
IV Semi-skilled	3%	31%	309
V Unskilled	1%	12%	115
Unclassified	0%	23%	93

workers being induced.

A possible explanation for the low induction rate among social class V mothers might have been the relatively low average birth weights of their babies. The proportion induced rose from 18 per cent of babies weighing less than $5\frac{1}{2}$ lb to 36 per cent of those weighing $9\frac{1}{2}$ lb or more (multiple births were excluded from this comparison). But this trend is due to differences at the two extremes. There was no trend in the proportion induced with baby's weight in the range $5\frac{1}{2}$ lb to 9 lb.

The average weight of the babies was similar, 7 lb 7 oz for the three middle-class groups, 7 lb 5 oz for the skilled manual and semi-skilled, and 7 lb 0 oz for the unskilled. Analysis of induction by baby's weight and social class showed that the only significant middle-class/working-class difference was among women whose babies weighed $7\frac{1}{2}$ lb or more. Among them, 20 per cent of the wives of non-manual workers were induced compared with 30 per cent of the wives of manual workers. However, the differences between the wives of men in unskilled jobs and those of other manual workers persisted for the four broad groups (although it was not significant for one of the four). The figures are in *Table 13*.

The social class differences cannot be explained by the type of hospital at which the babies were born, nor by variations in estimated length of gestation.

Another hypothesis for the social class variations related to women's certainty about the date of their last monthly period. The proportion who could not give a date or month for that was 11 per cent of the middle-class mothers, 16 per cent of those married to skilled or semi-

Table 13 Inductions by social class and baby's weight

Social class	Proportion induced							
	Baby's weight							
	Under 6½ lb		6½ lb < 7 lb		7 lb < 7½ lb		7½ lb or more	
I Professional	14%	(44)	21%	(29)	22%	(36)	21%	(80)
II Intermediate	18%	(60)	24%	(41)	27%	(79)	19%	(179)
III Skilled {Non-manual	20%	(30)	15%	(39)	29%	(52)	21%	(111)
{Manual	23%	(169)	23%	(148)	25%	(156)	30%	(362)
IV Semi-skilled	29%	(62)	31%	(58)	24%	(49)	36%	(132)
V Unskilled	11%	(27)	9%	(23)	13%	(24)	13%	(38)
	22%	(408)	22%	(354)	25%	(416)	26%	(942)

Table 14 Inductions by social class and hospitalization during pregnancy

Social class	Proportion admitted to hospital during pregnancy	Proportion induced among	
		Those admitted to hospital during pregnancy	Those not admitted to hospital during pregnancy
I Professional	23%	34% (44)	17% (150)
II Intermediate	21%	35% (75)	17% (292)
III Skilled {Non-manual	21%	34% (50)	17% (189)
{Manual	22%	44% (190)	21% (662)
IV Semi-skilled	25%	42% (77)	28% (232)
V Unskilled	14%	19%* (16)	11% (99)
Unclassified	20%	33%* (18)	20% (75)

* Based on less than twenty cases.

skilled manual workers, and 22 per cent of those married to unskilled workers. However, certainty about L M P was not related to induction.

Yet another possibility was that mothers in social class V were less exposed to the chance of induction because they received less intense ante-natal care. They were less likely to be admitted to hospital during pregnancy – 14 per cent of them were admitted compared with 23 per cent of other working-class mothers and 21 per cent of middle-class ones.[6] Induction was clearly related to previous admission: 39 per cent of those who had been admitted were induced, compared with 20 per cent of other mothers.

However, as the data in *Table 14* show, the induction rate in social class V was still relatively low both for those who were and for those who were not admitted to hospital during their pregnancy.

The wide variation in induction rates between the twenty-four study areas is another possible source of class variation, but there was no indication that these area differences contributed to the social class ones. So the puzzle about the social class differences remains.

Pregnancy

Women who were induced had had a more difficult pregnancy than those who went into labour spontaneously. Twenty-six per cent of the former, 18 per cent of the latter described it as 'rather difficult' or 'very difficult'.[7] And more of the induced reported problems of gaining too much weight (36 per cent compared with 28 per cent), high blood pressure or toxaemia (35 per cent against 17 per cent), swollen ankles (49 per cent and 40 per cent), the baby not growing fast enough (11 per cent and 6 per cent), and trouble sleeping (56 per cent and 51 per cent). There were no differences in the other fifteen symptoms they were asked about (feeling sick, being sick, headaches, nerves or depression, undue tiredness, vaginal bleeding, vaginal discharge, backache, trouble with water or kidneys, varicose veins, constipation, piles, lack of sexual feeling, painful or uncomfortable intercourse, indigestion or heartburn).

Rather more of those who were induced than of other mothers said they had had some worries or anxieties while they were pregnant:[8] 62 per cent compared with 57 per cent of other mothers. This may well be related to their additional symptoms and to the greater proportion who were admitted to hospital.

If anything, those who were induced went for their first ante-natal

[6] Mothers were asked: 'Did you have to go into hospital as an in-patient at any stage during your pregnancy?' Both interviewers and coders were instructed *not* to include admissions when they were already in labour or ones where they came in just before they were induced or had a Caesarean.

[7] They were asked: 'Would you say you had: a very easy pregnancy, a fairly easy pregnancy, a rather difficult pregnancy, or a very difficult pregnancy?'

[8] They were asked: 'Did you have any worries or anxieties while you were pregnant – about the baby or about having the baby?'

visit rather earlier than the others: a fifth of them left it until they were at least sixteen weeks pregnant compared with a quarter of the others. This ties in with the small proportion of social class V mothers who were induced, since a relatively high proportion of them, 35 per cent, left it sixteen weeks or more before their first ante-natal. But it does not relate to the other social class difference, since few, 20 per cent, of the middle class left it so late compared with 25 per cent in the other working-class (excluding V) groups. Slightly more of the induced went to hospital for some of their ante-natal care (78 per cent against 72 per cent), and rather fewer got some of this care from their general practitioner (78 per cent against 84 per cent). There was no difference in the proportion who had attended ante-natal classes.

Reasons for induction

Women whose labours were induced were asked why they thought it had been done.[9] All except 3 per cent gave some 'medical' reason, the most common ones being that they were overdue (55 per cent) that 'they' were worried about the baby (28 per cent), or that the mother had high blood pressure or toxaemia (27 per cent). Many mothers gave more than one reason, and some of the overlaps are indicated in Table 15.

Sixteen per cent of the women who were induced said that this was partly because they had wanted it, but only seven, 1 per cent, gave this as the only reason: 'He knew I was fed up and he knew I'd been in a lot of pain. I think he was just feeling kind. I must have been nearly ready or he would not have done it.'

Eleven per cent thought it was done so that the baby would be born at a convenient time, and a further 4 per cent were uncertain whether that was a reason. Nearly half these women, 5 per cent of those having inductions, thought it was for the convenience of both the mother and the hospital, 4 per cent that it was for the convenience of the hospital only, and 2 per cent for the mother.

---

[9] They were asked: 'What reasons, if any, did the doctor give why you should be induced?' 'So do you think it was because: you wanted it, you were overdue, you had high blood pressure, they thought the baby was getting too big, they were worried about the baby, you had rhesus negative blood, you had a long journey to hospital, the baby might come on its own too quickly for you to get to hospital, so that the baby would be born at a convenient time, so you could have an epidural. Were there any other reasons?'

Table 15   Mothers' perceptions of reasons for induction

	%
Medical	
Overdue	55 ⎫ 60
They thought the baby was getting too big	16 ⎭ ⎫ 40
They were worried about the baby	28 ⎭
Mother had high blood pressure or toxaemia	27
Rhesus incompatibility	9
Uncertain if medical reason	3
No medical reason	3
Other reasons	
Mother wanted it	16
So that baby would be born at convenient time	11
Possibly for baby to be born at convenient time	4
Mother had long journey to hospital	2
Baby might be born too quickly for mother to get to hospital	2
So mother could have an epidural	2
Number of mothers who were induced* (= 100%)	527

* Includes eleven for whom it was uncertain whether or not they were induced.

Some comments from those who thought it was for the convenience of the hospital only were: 'I went on a Tuesday morning and there wasn't anyone else in the induction unit at the time so they thought I might as well go straight in'; 'I would have preferred not to be induced. I think it was more convenient for them because of the rhesus factor – they wanted to be sure I was in hospital'; 'My husband had been talking to the doctor and he said I didn't want to be induced. Anyway, they took me in and broke my waters and put me on a drip, even though I didn't want it. I felt as though I'd been ganged up against.'

Data from medical records about the reason for induction were available for all of the forty-one patients reported by the doctors as having had an induction.[10] Over half of these, 66 per cent, were said to

[10]   The person extracting the data was asked to indicate which of the following reasons applied: 'Mother passed EDD, mother had raised blood pressure or toxaemia, to avoid disproportion, rhesus incompatibility, other high risk fetal factors, possibility of precipitate labour, mother had long journey to hospital, to ensure availability of optimum care, mother wanted it, other reason (to be written in)'.

be past the expected date of delivery (the EDD), for 12 per cent high blood pressure or toxaemia was recorded, and, in two instances, 5 per cent, a reason for induction was to ensure the availability of optimum care. There were a variety of other recorded reasons: 'Twin pregnancy at term'; 'Dates quite uncertain. Patient had had no period for two years. We estimated she was about term and so induced.' For over half, 56 per cent, of these patients, the sole reason given for inducing was that the mother was past her EDD. Only a fifth of the mothers who were induced gave 'overdue' as the only reason. The extent to which they were overdue is shown in *Table 16*.[11]

Table 16   Stage at which overdue mothers were induced

Number of days after EDD	Reports by mothers		Data from doctors	
	All those overdue	Those for whom being overdue was sole reason	All those past EDD	Those for whom this was sole reason
	%	%	%	%
1–6	12	4	8	—
7, 8, 9	21	19	23	23
10, 11, 12	22	29	46	50
13, 14, 15	32	38	15	18
16–20	6	6	8	9
21 or more	7	4	—	—
Number of inductions (= 100%)	283	97	26	22

Whereas the data from the mothers indicated that just over half of the inductions carried out because the mother was past her EDD were done within twelve days of the EDD, the information from the medical records suggests this proportion may be nearer three-quarters.

Mothers were also asked how many weeks pregnant they were when the baby was born. (In the sub-sample, the correlation between the mothers' estimates of this and the doctors' estimates of gestational age was + 0.76.) Analyses suggest that nearly a third of the induced births occurred in the forty-second week or later, two-thirds in the thirty-

---

[11] Mothers were asked how overdue they were reckoned to be at the time of the induction. The question for doctors was phrased differently: 'When did the birth occur in relation to the EDD?'

Table 17   Induction and gestational age

Weeks pregnant when baby born	Elective Caesarean section	Induced	Started spon- taneously	All live births	Proportion induced*	
	%	%	%	%		
Less than 36	2	1	2	2	13%	(45)
36	13	1	2	2	12%	(42)
37	2	2	5	4	10%	(86)
38	23	7	9	8	20%	(179)
39	31	12	16	15	18%	(328)
40	15	23	35	32	18%	(671)
41	8	24	20	21	28%	(437)
42	6	24	9	13	46%	(262)
43	—	4	1	2	51%	(37)
44	—	1	}1	}1	}42%	(26)
45 or more	—	1				
Number of mothers *(= 100%)*	48	508	1557	2125		

* Figures in brackets are the numbers on which the percentages are based (= 100%).

eighth to forty-first weeks (see *Table 17*). Looking at the proportion of births that were induced, shown in the last column, this was around one in eight of births occurring in or before the thirty-seventh week, one in five of those in the thirty-eighth, thirty-ninth, and fortieth weeks, rising to almost half of those in the forty-second week or later.

The mothers' perceptions about the reason for induction were related to gestational age. The proportion induced because of high blood pressure declined from over half, 54 per cent, of those induced before the fortieth week to 11 per cent of those induced in the forty-second week or later, while the proportion induced because they were thought to be overdue rose from 6 per cent to 95 per cent.

Timing of induced births

The days of the week on which different types of births occurred are shown in *Table 18*. Elective Caesarean sections were most likely to occur on Mondays and relatively few of these were done at week ends. Comparatively few induced births were delivered on a Sunday, but apart from this they were relatively evenly distributed over the other six days. Surprisingly, births resulting from spontaneous labours were *not* evenly distributed: a smaller proportion than expected occurred on Saturday and a relatively high proportion on Wednesdays. Possibly

Table 18 Days of week on which different types of birth occurred

	Elective Caesarean section	Induced	Spontaneous start	All births*
	%	%	%	%
Monday	25	13	14	14
Tuesday	8	19	14	15
Wednesday	19	15	17	16
Thursday	19	17	14	15
Friday	17	15	16	16
Saturday	6	15	12	12
Sunday	6	6	13	12
Number of births (= 100%)	48	522	1599	2182

* Includes thirteen births that may have been induced or spontaneous.

Table 19 Time of day at which spontaneous and induced births were delivered

	Induced	Spontaneous start
	%	%
Midnight < 3 a.m.	7	10
3 a.m. < 6 a.m.	3	13
6 a.m. < 9 a.m.	3	13
9 a.m. < 12 noon	5	13
Noon < 3 p.m.	17	11
3 p.m. < 6 p.m.	27	14
6 p.m. < 9 p.m.	22	14
9 p.m. < midnight	16	12
Number of births (= 100%)	518	1592

some women prefer to have their babies during the week rather than at weekends, and 23 per cent of those whose labours started spontaneously said there was something that which happened to them or which they did before they went into labour that they thought might have helped to bring it on.

Acceleration, as well as induction, may affect the timing of birth, but it would seem likely that this would have a greater influence on the time of the day rather than the day of the week. However, *Table 19* suggests that labours that started spontaneously, even though some of them were subsequently accelerated, resulted in births spread fairly evenly throughout the twenty-four hours, whereas those resulting from induced labours were more frequently delivered between 3 p.m. and midnight. This differs from the finding of Cole, Howie, and Macnaughton (1975) that the hour of delivery was similar in the induced and in their control group. Data from *British Births 1970* (Chamberlain *et al.* 1975: 114) show a relatively high proportion of all deliveries occurring between 5 p.m. and midnight.

So half, 49 per cent, of the induced births on this study occurred during normal working hours (9 a.m. to 6 p.m.) compared with 38 per cent of the other births. There was also an excess of evening births among the induced and a relative dearth between midnight and noon.

Conclusions

The information from this study throws some doubt on the HIPE figures about induction. It seems likely that the proportion of induced labours is between a quarter and a third rather than two-fifths. The proportion in which oxytocin or prostaglandins are used to start or to accelerate or augment labour will be rather higher.

Although labours that are induced result in fewer deliveries at weekends or in the early hours of the morning, there is little evidence from this study that inductions are often done mainly for the convenience of the hospital or staff.

At the same time there is no indication of a general policy of induction related to risk factors and associated with characteristics of the mothers, while institutional attributes—the size of hospital, the type of hospital, being a private or NHS patient, the area and the hospital itself—were all related to induction.

The observation that a comparatively small proportion of women in social class V were induced merits further research. A 'small-for-dates' fetus is commonly regarded as a major indication for induction and is more likely to occur among these women. And there is clear evidence that social class V women were less often admitted to hospital during pregnancy than other mothers.

One group of women who might have been particularly likely to have an induction because of various high risk factors are those who had a still birth. These are considered in the next chapter.

3 Still birth and induction

Conditions which cause still birth can be a reason for induction. Diagnoses of toxaemia or placental insufficiency may lead doctors to induce labour in an attempt to save the baby. In other instances, if anencephaly or other gross malformations which cause still births are diagnosed ante-natally, doctors may decide to induce labour as there seems little point in prolonging pregnancy. This also applies when the fetus is known to have died. For these reasons, a study of induction would have been incomplete if it had not included a sample of still births.

In order to get adequate numbers of still births to consider as a separate group, a relatively high proportion of still births was included in the study. In the initial sample, 240 still births were included compared with 2,400 live births, so 9.1 per cent of the total sample were still births. Among those who were interviewed, the proportion was somewhat lower, 8.2 per cent, because more of the women who had had a still birth refused or could not be contacted. In England in 1975, there were 1.0 still births per 100 live and still births.

In this chapter, the proportions of inductions are considered in relation to the cause of the still birth. After that, various other aspects of the women's experience during pregnancy and delivery are compared with women who had a live birth. Differences that emerge are examined in relation to whether or not the labour was induced.

As expected, a relatively high proportion of the women who had a still birth were thirty-five or more (11 per cent compared with 5 per cent of those who had a live birth), were having their first pregnancy

(48 per cent against 37 per cent), and had had four or more previous pregnancies (6 per cent against 2 per cent). Eight per cent had had an earlier still birth compared with 2 per cent of those who had a live birth.

Inductions and cause of still birth

Labour was induced for over a third, 36 per cent, of the women who had a still birth. This is higher than the proportion for live births, 24 per cent. The proportion varied considerably in relation to the cause of the still birth, as can be seen from *Table 20*.[1]

Table 20   Inductions by cause of still birth

Main cause	Proportion having elective Caesarean section	Proportion induced	Number of still births (= 100%)
Toxaemia of pregnancy	4%	52%	23
Difficult labour and other complications of pregnancy and childbirth	6%*	28%*	18
Placenta praevia, etc.	5%*	16%*	19
Other conditions of placenta	0%	38%	21
Conditions of umbilical cord	0%*	41%*	17
Congenital abnormalities of the nervous system	0%	55%	38
Anoxic and hypoxic conditions, immaturity, maceration, and unknown causes	0%	20%	44
Other conditions	6%*	38%*	16
All still births	2%	36%	196

* Based on less than twenty cases.

The proportion of inductions was relatively high, over half, for still births due to toxaemia or resulting from congenital abnormalities of the nervous system. The proportion of elective Caesarean sections was similar for still births and live births.

For 109, 56 per cent, of the still births information was obtained

[1] For details about the classification of cause of still births and a comparison with national statistics, see *Appendix IV*.

from medical records. The data about induction from the records tallied with the interview information from the mother in 86 per cent of cases. Doctors also reported a higher (although insignificant) pro-portion of inductions among the still births than among the live births, but no increase in Caesarean sections.

Reasons for the induction of still births recorded in the medical records were intrauterine death in two-fifths of the cases, and anencephaly or other fetal abnormality for a fifth. Three out of forty-one were induced because the mother was past the expected date of delivery.

The pregnancy and ante-natal care

Women who had a still birth were more likely than mothers who had a live baby to describe their pregnancy as difficult: 35 per cent compared with 19 per cent. The various symptoms they reported during pregnancy are shown in *Table 21*.

The first thing that strikes one is the number of symptoms associated with pregnancy: an average of 7.2 for women who had a live birth and 7.9 for those who had a still birth. For both groups the symptom that was said to have bothered them most was indigestion or heartburn. Many more of those who had a still birth reported that they had problems because the baby was not growing fast enough and that they had high blood pressure or toxaemia. They were also more likely to report headaches, vaginal bleeding, and 'other symptoms'; they less often reported trouble sleeping. This last difference probably arose because those who had still births had smaller babies: three-fifths of their babies were under $5\frac{1}{2}$ lb compared with 5 per cent of the live births.[2] Increasing physical discomfort associated with a heavy fetus probably interferes with sleep. Among those who had a live birth the proportion reporting trouble with sleeping rose from 43 per cent of those whose babies weighed less than $5\frac{1}{2}$ lb to 72 per cent of those whose babies weighed $9\frac{1}{2}$ lb or more.

Over a third, 37 per cent, of those who had a still birth had been admitted to hospital as an in-patient during their pregnancy com-pared with less than a quarter, 22 per cent, of those who had a live baby. In view of these different experiences it is not surprising that

[2] Almost a third of the women who had a still birth did not give us information about the weight, but data from medical records also indicate that two-thirds of the still births weighed less than $5\frac{1}{2}$ lb.

Table 21   Symptoms during pregnancy

	Live birth	Still birth	Significance of difference
	%	%	
Feeling sick	66	65	NS
Actually being sick	46	49	NS
Gaining too much weight	30	30	NS
High blood pressure or toxaemia	22	36	< .001
Headaches	24	32	< .05
Nerves or depression	33	38	NS
Swollen ankles	43	46	NS
Undue tiredness	54	57	NS
Vaginal bleeding	13	19	< .05
Vaginal discharge	34	39	NS
Backache	58	55	NS
Trouble sleeping	52	44	< .05
Trouble with water or kidneys	19	25	NS
The baby not growing fast enough	7	31	< .001
Varicose veins	15	15	NS
Constipation	35	32	NS
Piles	24	21	NS
Lack of sexual feeling	27	29	NS
Painful or uncomfortable intercourse	21	23	NS
Indigestion or heartburn	67	64	NS
Other symptoms	22	31	< .01
No symptoms	3	2	NS

Number of women (= 100%) 2182   196

more of those who had a still birth said they had been worried or anxious about the baby during their pregnancy. But the difference was not great: 50 per cent compared with 41 per cent of those who had a live birth. There was no difference in the proportion expressing anxiety about having the baby: nearly a quarter. Over two-fifths who said they had some worries during pregnancy said they had not discussed these anxieties with a doctor, midwife, nurse, or anyone like that. This did not differ significantly between those who had a still birth and those who had a live birth, but the proportion who described the person they had talked to as 'not very helpful' was much higher for those who had a still birth, 29 per cent, compared with 11 per cent of those who had a live birth.

Some felt they had been reassured inappropriately: ' "There's nothing to worry about," they kept saying. They just didn't say any more'; 'They said that I was worrying unnecessarily. It's easy to tell someone not to worry.' Some particular anxieties they had been unable to discuss were: 'I was on a drug when I fell for the baby. I couldn't discuss it with anyone properly. I asked them if it could harm the baby but they never explained it to put your mind at rest. The only thing they said it would do was to make the baby fat.'

'I did mention that I thought it [the baby] was not growing fast enough. He said it felt all right – the uterus was the right height. They said it was normal at the end of pregnancy for the movements to be less. My other two babies were small and I mentioned this to him, but he took no notice. He should have checked me himself. He could have done other tests.'

The stage at which women had first attended for ante-natal care was similar for those who had still births and those who had live births, and the sources of their ante-natal care were also similar.[3] Three had had no ante-natal care. One of these was an undiagnosed pregnancy. Another had not consulted a doctor at all:

'I thought my periods had stopped because of the nervous state I was in. When I did realize, I was six months gone and was very upset at the thought of having another baby as my husband and I had separated by then. I was taken into hospital as an emergency when I went into labour.'

The third had seen her doctor first when she was eight weeks pregnant but 'I went away, for he said it was the change of life'. She then went at three months and arranged to have the birth in a maternity home, but she had not had any ante-natal care because: 'I didn't want them mucking me about – mithering about. I don't get on with the health visitor and I had just lost another, see' (aged 35 to 39 with five children and had had a still birth three years previously).

Length of pregnancy

One very large difference between the still births and the live births

---

[3] This remains true when only those having their first pregnancy are compared.

Table 22   Length of pregnancy

Weeks	Live birth	Still birth	Estimated number of still births per 1,000 live and still births
	%	%	
Less than 36	2	43	175
36	2	11	56
37	4	9	23
38	8	8	9
39	15	8	6
40	32	11	4
41	21	4	2
42	13	4	3
43	2	1	} 7
44 or more	1	1	
Number of women (= *100%*)	2125	194	10

was the length of the pregnancy at the time of delivery.[4]

Slightly over half, 54 per cent, of the still births occurred when the women estimated they were thirty-six weeks or less pregnant. Only 4 per cent of the live births occurred so early on. Although only a small proportion of the still births occurred in the forty-third week or later, estimates of the still-birth rate dropped from 175 per 1,000 for pregnancies ending before the thirty-sixth week to two for those ending in the forty-first week, and then rose after that. But these figures indicate that an increase in intervention on or after term can have relatively little effect on the still-birth rate since so few still births occur at that stage.

Analysis by the cause of the still birth showed that a relatively high proportion of those attributed to toxaemia of pregnancy occurred when the woman was less than thirty-six weeks pregnant: 70 per cent compared with 40 per cent of other still births.

Related to this, the proportion of inductions was 36 per cent among still births occurring when the woman was less than forty weeks pregnant, fell to 14 per cent among those occurring during the fortieth

[4] Among the 109 still births for which data were available from medical records, the correlation between the women's and the doctors' estimates was 0.82.

week, and rose to 56 per cent among the few still births that occurred later in pregnancy. This pattern is different from the one found among live births and shown in the previous chapter. For them the proportion of inductions increased fairly steadily with length of gestation and did not show any marked trough around the fortieth week.

Labour

There was no difference between women having a live or still birth in the proportion (four-fifths) who said they were given something to relieve their pain during labour, but the type of analgesic they were given was different. A higher proportion of those who had a still birth were given an epidural: 10 per cent compared with 5 per cent of those who had a live birth; fewer were given something to inhale, 39 per cent against 51 per cent; and a smaller proportion said they were given pethidine, 20 per cent compared with 30 per cent. There was no difference in the proportion (over a third) who were given something but did not know what it was. Their reactions to the anaesthetics they were given (or not given) were similar in most ways.[5]

Two-thirds of those who had a still birth said the nurses and midwives had been 'very helpful' during their labour.[6] Rather more, three-quarters, of those who had a live birth felt this, but of course those assessments were made retrospectively and may have been influenced by the outcome. The women in the two groups identified very similar types of people as being the greatest help to them during the first stages of their labour: over a third of both groups said it was the nurses or midwives, three-tenths that it was their husbands. Husbands were as likely to have been there at some stage of the labour for those having still births as for those having live births, but they were less likely to have been present at the delivery – for 11 per cent of the still births, 36 per cent of the live births. However, when the women whose husbands were not with them 'from beginning to end' were asked if they would have liked him to be there, or to be there for longer, rather fewer of those having a still birth said they would have liked this – 42 per cent compared with 50 per cent of those who had a live baby. So for one reason or another just over a third of those having a

---

[5] Three per cent of those who had a still birth compared with 7 per cent of those who had a live birth said they would rather have not been given anything.

[6] 'Would you describe the nurses and midwives during your labour as very helpful, fairly helpful, not very helpful?'

still birth did not have the company and support of their husbands when they would have liked it, and two-fifths of this group said they did not think the hospital would have agreed to this. A further third were uncertain:

'I suppose if we'd really insisted they might have agreed, but they didn't want him to see it because they were frightened of him actually seeing the baby because she was in such a very bad state. They wouldn't let me see either. They put a cloth over my legs.' (The baby was anencephalic.)

A relatively high proportion of those who had a still birth were unable to estimate the length of the first stage of their labour: 15 per cent said they could not do so compared with 3 per cent of those who had a live birth. Among those who could estimate it there were no significant differences. If anything, a somewhat smaller proportion of those who had had a still birth said it lasted less than six hours: 32 per cent compared with 38 per cent of those with a live birth. Differences in the length of time they said they had experienced had pain during their labour[7] were also equivocal – a higher proportion of those who had a still birth than of those who had a live birth said not at all (17 per cent against 10 per cent) – but the proportions having bad pain for less than two hours were 40 per cent and 49 per cent in the two groups.

Over half, 52 per cent, of those who had a still birth said they were worried or anxious during their labour compared with less than a third of those who had a live birth. But of course this means that most of those who were worried had a live baby. Just over half those who were worried had discussed their anxieties with someone at the time, but nearly half had not done so. Nurses, doctors, and their husband were the people they had most often talked to. Half of those who had a still birth said the person they had talked to had been very helpful, but over a quarter described them as 'not very helpful'.[8] Doctors and nurses were more often categorized in this last way than husbands (46 per cent against 6 per cent).

'I could not communicate with anyone – not like you. They were so unsympathetic and not even the Asian nurses would talk to me.'
                    (An Asian woman, interviewed with an interpreter)

'I felt something was very wrong – they brushed it off. I'd rather

[7] 'For how long, if at all, during your labour would you say you had bad pain?'
[8] This proportion did not differ significantly from those who had a live birth.

they'd told me, but obviously they didn't want to frighten me.'

'I was concerned about the baby being so small. I asked the doctor when I was in labour what the baby's chances were and he said, "very good", but before I started pushing down they couldn't hear the baby's heartbeat. They were so busy they couldn't stay with me all the time, I had to keep ringing for them. When I felt I wanted to bear down I rang for the midwife and she tried to get the baby's heartbeat but she couldn't, so she "bleeped" for the doctor, but by the time he came it was born. I just felt the doctor had raised my hopes too high during labour.'

Some reasons they gave for not discussing their anxieties were:

'There was no-one there. They just popped in and out, that was all.'

'They were busy and I felt they were doing their best and it was just one of those things I had to endure.'

'I knew there was something wrong and I just wanted to get it over with.'

'I just didn't like talking about it. They would only have said it wasn't [dead] or not to worry.'

There was no difference between those who had had still births and those who had had a live birth in the proportion who said they were left alone at some stage during their labour (over two-fifths of both groups said this). But rather more of those who had had a live birth said they did not mind being left alone: 31 per cent compared with 24 per cent.

The only difference in the symptoms they reported during their labour was that rather more of those who had a still birth said they vomited: 26 per cent against 20 per cent – but since they were asked about several symptoms, such a difference might occur by chance.

All in all, the picture that emerges is of surprisingly similar assessments of their experience during labour. The totally different outcome seems to have coloured the women's retrospective descriptions of their labour very little. The few differences may well be real ones: those who had a still birth having longer first stages, more often being given an epidural, more of them preferring not to be left alone, and more finding nurses and midwives unhelpful.

Delivery

Similar proportions of still and live births took place outside hospital and nursing homes but fewer still births, 2 per cent, were initially booked for home delivery, compared with 5 per cent of live births. Three of the still births that occurred at home just did not make it to the hospital, and one was an undiagnosed pregnancy. 'I never knew I was pregnant until the day I lost it. The doctor said I was going through the change. I disputed that – I was too young [thirty-six] – but he said I wasn't. He did ask me if I thought I was pregnant and I said no.' A high proportion of the women who had still births did not have it in the place that was arranged: 23 per cent compared with 11 per cent of those who had a live birth. Much of this transference was from one hospital to another, which probably explains why less than 1 per cent of the still births occurred in a general practitioner hospital or maternity home compared with 5 per cent of live births.

Those who had a still birth were *less* likely to have an emergency Caesarean section: 1.6 per cent of them did so, against 3.7 per cent of those who had a live birth. There was no indication of any difference in the proportion of assisted deliveries,[9] but more of those who had a still birth said they did not know whether any instruments were used to help the baby out: 19 per cent compared with 3 per cent of those who had a live birth. In addition, fewer knew whether the baby came out head first, or was a breech, or what: 76 per cent compared with 99 per cent. But among those who did know there were many more breech deliveries among the still births: 24 per cent against 3 per cent. (Even if none of those who did not know had a breech delivery, the difference would still be very considerable, 18 per cent against 3 per cent.) Episiotomy[10] was less often reported by those who had a still birth: 23 per cent against 49 per cent. And only a third of those who had a still birth compared with over two-thirds of the others had stitches. Of course, the still-born babies were smaller.

More of the still births were delivered by a doctor, 34 per cent compared with 19 per cent, but women who had a still birth were no more or less likely than those having a live birth to say the consultant or general practitioner in charge of them was at the delivery. Data from the medical records, in *Table 23*, show that registrars were more likely to be involved in the delivery of still births, and midwives in training possibly less so.

As with live births, the majority of still births were delivered by midwives, and for two-thirds of these no other professional person was

---

[9] 'Were any instruments used to get the baby out?'
[10] 'Did they cut you at all?'

present. A qualified midwife or a doctor was there at all live or still births delivered by a midwife in training.

Table 23   The person who delivered the live or still birth (data from medical records)

	Live births	Still births
	%	%
Consultant	2	3
Registrar	7	22
House Officer or		
Senior House Officer	7	9
General practitioner	4	1
Medical student	3	—
Qualified midwife	60	55
Midwife in training	16	8
Other	1	2
Number of vaginal		
deliveries (= 100%)	117	102

Aftercare in hospital

Women who had a still birth stayed in hospital for a relatively short time after the delivery compared with those who had a live birth. A third of them stayed less than two days and nearly three-quarters were out within four days. Corresponding proportions for those who had a live birth were one in fifteen leaving within two days, and one-third within four days. At the other end of the scale, 6 per cent of those who had a still birth and 19 per cent of those who had a live birth stayed in ten days or longer. The mothers' assessments of their length of stay were more similar, just over three-fifths of each group thought it about right, but only 3 per cent of those who had a still birth compared with 8 per cent of those who had a live one would have preferred to stay in longer. Possibly because of the shorter length of stay, a smaller proportion of those who had a still birth reported problems or complications for themselves while they were in hospital and after the birth: 31 per cent against 37 per cent of those who had a live birth.[11]

A quarter of those who had a still birth and a tenth of the others said

[11] A difference that might have occurred by chance.

that other people's babies had disturbed or irritated them a lot while they were in hospital. The wording of this question was probably more appropriate for those who had a live birth, as some of the comments from those who had a still birth suggest: 'When I heard them crying I had a little weep to myself. I remember one lunchtime a woman came in and said, "Oh, my little lad has been a sod". I thought how I wished I could say that about mine'; 'That's why I wanted to come out. I was in a little room but it was beside where the mothers and babies were and I had to go through there to go to the toilet. I felt they were all looking at me and feeling sorry for me. I couldn't bear that.'

There was no difference between those having live and still births in their descriptions of their comfort[12] during the time they were in hospital, nor for those who had stitches in their assessment of the pain and discomfort caused by the stitches. Neither did they differ in their rating of how well they slept in hospital. More of those who had had a still birth were offered or given sleeping pills, 82 per cent compared with 75 per cent of those who had a live birth; fewer asked for them, 3 per cent against 6 per cent; and more took them, 75 per cent compared with 62 per cent.

When asked if they had felt weepy at all while they were in hospital, 83 per cent of those who had a still birth and 55 per cent of those with a live birth said they had done so. Some comments from those with still births were: 'I kept thinking about it and I was always expecting them to bring it through the door'; '. . . all for nothing. No-one can understand the emptiness'; 'When my husband came in I broke down. I couldn't cry straight away. I think I was a bit shocked when I saw it lying there.' A few had not cried until they got home: 'On the Tuesday when I came home, I heard a baby crying and it broke my heart – but while I was in hospital I think I tried to put a brave face on it'; 'I didn't, not until I came home and had to see everyone. In hospital I felt numb.'

Care at home

Women who had had a still birth more often reported that when they got home they had been given help by their mother (56 per cent against 49 per cent), and a sister or a sister-in-law (36 per cent against 27 per cent). There was no difference in the proportion receiving help

[12] 'During that time would you say you were very comfortable, fairly comfortable, or uncomfortable?'

from their mothers-in-law, other relatives, or friends and neighbours, and their views on who had helped them most were similar. One per cent in each group had had the aid of a local authority home help.

Husbands whose wives had had a still birth were less likely to take time off as a holiday to look after their wives (40 per cent against 48 per cent), more likely to take time off without pay (10 per cent against 6 per cent), and more likely to be given time off (11 per cent against 3 per cent).

Only 3 per cent of those women who had a still birth said they would have liked more help compared with 17 per cent of those who had a live birth, but just over a quarter of each group said they had some difficulties or problems when they got home. Some descriptions of their emotional problems by those who had had a still birth were: 'The main problem is, when you lose a baby people treat you as though you hadn't had one. People would cross the street to avoid me'; 'My little boy – I became over-protective. My nerves were very bad. I was terrified to leave him out of my sight for fear he got killed, but I've adapted now and am more in control'; 'I felt empty, as though I'd left something. I felt a great loss as though something was missing'; 'It only hit me when I got home, when I saw all the baby's things.'

There were physical problems too – with bleeding, discharge, soreness, milk, urine, etc.: 'I had troubles with stitches and water. I never dropped back into place. I was depressed and couldn't sleep. I had to go on Valium'; 'Waiting for the milk to dry up – that was upsetting. When I had Jane they used to give tablets, but they don't now – and it did upset me emotionally a lot.' Sometimes they felt the services were not as helpful as they might have been:

> 'I couldn't pass urine, but the doctor said I would eventually go back. It was the pipe that had stretched when I had the baby. I thought it was bad I didn't see the gynaecologist I was supposed to be under. Once the baby had died he didn't see me any more.'

Those who had had a still birth were asked: 'Since you got home, who have you talked to mainly about your experience?', and then whom they had found most helpful. Their replies are shown in *Table 24*, alongside the replies of those who had had a live birth to questions about whom they had talked to about having the baby and looking after the baby.

Three-quarters of the women who had had a still birth discussed their experience with their husband, and nearly half said they had

Table 24   Discussions about their experience

	Live births		Still births	
	Discussion about having the baby and about looking after the baby		Discussions about their experience	
	Talked to mainly	Most helpful	Talked to mainly	Most helpful
	%	%	%	%
Husband	55	25	74	45
Mother	34	15	40	9
Mother-in-law	12	3	14	2
Sister or sister-in-law	17	6	14	2
Other relatives	5	1	8	1
Friends or neighbours	37	15	36	10
Health visitor	20	15	11	2
Nurse or midwife	13	5	18	8
Doctor	7	3	25	5
Other person	2	1	5	1
No-one	9	11	11	15
Number of women (= 100%)	2177	2096	194	173

found him the most helpful person to talk to. But one in seven had not had any discussions they thought helpful. Discussions with mothers and health visitors about live babies proved more helpful than those about still births. Some of those who had had a still birth described ways in which their mothers had not been altogether helpful:

'I felt my mother was a problem sometimes being here. I wanted to do things and couldn't. My mother was really upset and my husband told her only to do the things I wanted and she took this to the letter. If I had been here on my own I think I could have had a really good cry.'

'My mother wanted to rule the house, and she did mean well, but she took over completely, and this upset me. She wasn't going to come originally, my husband was going to look after us. She just packed her bags and left poor Dad – he didn't have a say – and over she came.'

'It was all a bit tight because they all wanted to do things. My mother was upset. But really, they were sorry for themselves, not for me. My mother wanted sympathy herself.'

More of those who had a still birth had talked to a doctor about their experience, but relatively few said these discussions had been the most helpful ones they had had. A quarter of those who had had a still birth (compared with a tenth of those with a live baby) said they would have liked to talk to someone else about their experience, and the type of person they most frequently mentioned in this connection was a doctor – nearly a fifth of all those who had had a still birth would have welcomed some or more opportunity to discuss their experience with a doctor. Nine out of ten of them had seen their general practitioner since they had left hospital, and he had visited nearly three-fifths of them at home: three-fifths of those who had seen him described him as 'very helpful', a fifth as 'helpful', and another fifth as 'not very helpful'.

Those who had had a live birth were as likely to have seen their general practitioner, much more likely to have seen a health visitor (96 per cent of them had done so, 47 per cent of those who had had a still birth), but rather less likely to have seen a nurse or midwife since leaving hospital (71 per cent against 85 per cent). Among those who had had a still birth, 74 per cent described their contact with a nurse or midwife as 'very helpful' compared with only 43 per cent who felt this about their contact with a health visitor. Mothers with live babies were also more likely to find their contacts with nurses or midwives very helpful than those with health visitors (68 per cent compared with 60 per cent), but more of them than of those who had a still birth said that the health visitor had been very helpful (60 per cent against 43 per cent).

When asked to assess their health since they got home, there was no significant difference between those who had a live and those who had a still birth (nearly half described it as very good), but when asked about various symptoms or problems,[13] slightly more of those who had had a still birth reported trouble with their breasts (26 per cent against 20 per cent) and many more reported nerves or depression (67 per cent against 45 per cent). But perhaps the most striking thing is that nearly half those who had had a live baby reported this. More of those who had had a live baby said they had suffered from undue tiredness (46 per cent compared with 37 per cent).

[13] 'Have you had any of these symptoms or problems: trouble with your breasts, bleeding, trouble passing water, constipation, nerves or depression, irritability, backache, undue tiredness, painful intercourse, anything else?'

Those who said they would like to have talked with someone else about their experience were more likely to report nerves or depression than those who did not want further discussion (86 per cent compared with 61 per cent), but the prevalence of nerves or depression also appeared relatively high among those who had discussed their experiences with their husband and found him 'the most helpful' (78 per cent against 55 per cent).

As deaths of infants and still births become less common, people may be less likely to develop skills in helping the unfortunate few who encounter these tragedies to cope with them. Relatives, and perhaps potential fathers and grandparents in particular, will feel a sense of loss and deprivation themselves. This study shows that they rally round to help with household tasks but sometimes fail to meet the emotional needs of the woman who may be feeling a sense of anxiety and shame as well as bereavement. A leader in the *Lancet* suggested that 'ordinary commonsense and kindliness are insufficient to meet the needs of these patients' (1977). It is clear that many professionals also lack necessary skills and insights, and a study by Bourne suggested that there is 'a strong reluctance of doctors to know, notice or remember anything about the patient who has had a still birth' (1968).

Information and choices

There was no difference between those who had still births and those who had live births in the proportion who would have liked more information about various aspects of their care – or who would have liked it earlier;[14] four-fifths would have liked more or earlier information. But the sorts of things they wanted more information about

---

[14] 'Thinking now about the information you were given. Would you have liked more information about any of these things – or would you have liked information about them earlier? What about: starting labour, process of labour, Caesarean operations, induction, epidural or spinal anaesthetic, other forms of pain relief, the pushing or second stage, actual delivery, being cut, being stitched, the afterbirth, the machines and gadgets they use, the baby's progress before labour (the baby's progress during labour, the baby's progress around delivery, the baby's progress in first two days, the baby's progress later on in hospital, breast feeding the baby, bottle feeding the baby, looking after the baby), your own progress after the baby was born, drying up the milk, getting rid of the stitches, anything else?' (Those who had had a still birth were not asked the section between brackets.)

varied. More of those who had had still births expressed dissatisfaction with the information they were given about the process of labour (22 per cent against 14 per cent), about Caesarean sections (28 per cent compared with 19 per cent), and about the baby's progress before labour (45 per cent compared with 32 per cent). Those who had had live births often wanted more information about the baby's progress after birth and about feeding the baby, but many of those who had still births expressed a desire for more information about why their baby died: 'I would like to know, for peace of mind. No-one has explained to me why.'

> 'With not knowing what actually happened to the baby – I'd prefer to be told the truth. No-one tells me anything. Yes, I've asked, and they said as soon as they cut the cord and baby died – but why no-one has explained. I'd feel better if I'd had it explained to me properly.'

> 'I never found what caused it. My doctor said "It's just one of those things" and I never got to see a consultant at the hospital.'

Some had tried unsuccessfully to get more information:

> 'The only thing I wanted to know at the time was why it didn't go normally, I'd never been told. I've asked twice. We were asked at____ if we wanted a post-mortem doing on the baby and we said yes. We've asked twice since if there's anything we should know. First time he said he'd had no results of it, the second time he said if there's anything we should know he'd let us know. Next time I asked him was when I went for the post-natal and he said he'd had nothing from the hospital, but not to worry, it was just one of those things. We asked him everything we could think of, such as smoking or being on the pill beforehand, and he said no. I wasn't satisfied. At____ they told my husband to 'phone them at the end of the week, or ask the doctor, and he asked him when he came here. He's told us nothing. I'd like to know if there was something I could have done I didn't do, or if it's something they gave me that caused it, or anything like that.'

Others had not done so: 'I didn't know enough about the cause – I'd like to have known more of the details. Perhaps they thought it best not to say any more, and I didn't ask.' Some were anxious about the implications for possible future pregnancies:

'Well, I'm scared in case it happens again. I mean, my own G. P. has explained a lot to me and is very resentful about the neglect I received at_____. Well, my G. P. has said next time I'm to have a special test that draws off fluid from around the waters, and they can tell the sex and whether or not the baby is normal, and if not there's no need to go the whole term – you just have an abortion – and there's a lot less distress.'

'I would like to have known the true facts of it happening again. The doctor the next day said it was a million to one chance, but my midwife said there was a tendency for it to happen again. I would have liked to know the truth. I know now, as we've seen a specialist about it. There is a test to prove if a baby is deformed – the same test they do for mongolism – and, if it's positive, they terminate the pregnancy. There is a one in twenty chance of it happening again. If the test is negative there is a one in 100 chance of it occurring. After I'd seen the specialist, I spoke to my G. P. about this. He didn't advise having the test done, because there was a slight chance that, even if the baby was normal, it would disturb it and I'd miscarry. He is rather soft, and said it would be better to have the baby anyway and, even if it was a mongol, not to worry as they can be very sweet and are very loyal, etc. This so upset me that I left the surgery in tears. It was the thing that most upset me after the birth.'

Some had not been informed about funeral arrangements:

'They didn't tell us about any arrangements – they didn't mention the baby at all. I thought they made all arrangements to see to him. After three days, I said to my husband, "I wonder where the baby is?" We asked, and they said he was waiting for us to bury him. So my husband had to go to the funeral shop and order a little box. Why didn't they tell us – we didn't know we had to do it. Suppose we hadn't asked – they would think we didn't care.'

And others wanted to know why certain things had not been done which they felt might have prevented the still birth:

'I used to say to my husband, "I reckon I can feel two lots of feet and hands" – only joking. There was never any mention of twins at all. I feel it was neglect they didn't discover the twins. I didn't know any history [of them] in my family, or my husband's, and we've found out since that there is in both families. I'd like to know why they didn't discover I was expecting two.'

'At the pregnancy beginning they should have given me tests for spina bifida – they didn't because they thought it couldn't happen again – but now they know it can happen again. I heard a nurse say I should have been given these tests at the beginning. They take a sample out of the womb, and though they can't tell what's the matter, they know if it's abnormal.'

'The only thing is, looking back, I think the doctor should have sent me to a clinic, or read a monitor to check the baby's heart more closely after I'd told him that I'd not felt the baby move for the last three days. I think he should have taken more notice. I pushed the point with him, but he didn't take any notice of me. If he had heard the baby's heart at that point, but had taken my opinion on it, perhaps a Caesarean at that stage might have saved the baby – I don't know.'

One woman wondered if it might have helped if she had seen the baby:

'Why the baby was born like she was. You don't take pills and you take care of yourself and then things go wrong. I tend to wish I'd have seen the baby, and then think if I had it would have been worse. I feel I'd like to talk to one of the doctors and try and find out more about it, but it wouldn't bring the baby back. Because it's you, you want to know why these things happen. I'd like to know the worst. Well, if she'd lived, what she would have been like, and would she eventually have been all right?'

While the proportion wanting more information was similar for those with live and for those with still births, the proportion who felt they had a choice about the type of care they were given was lower among those who had a still birth. Similar proportions, around 85 per cent, said they had been happy about the initial arrangements that were made about where they should have the baby, but only two-fifths of those who had a still birth felt they had had a choice about this compared with half of those who had a live birth. And, among those who were induced, fewer of those who had a still birth felt they could have refused it (34 per cent compared with 54 per cent of those who had a live birth), and fewer still felt they had a choice about it (17 per cent against 34 per cent). But, as will be shown later, feelings about choice were related to the reason for the induction.

Had their experience made them any more or less anxious to take decisions for themselves in the future, or influenced their preferences for types of treatment in future pregnancies? There was no evidence that it had done so. There was no difference between those who had live or still births in the proportions who would prefer a doctor to take a decision without consultation or to explain and let the patient choose, nor in their preferences for an induction, an epidural, or a home birth at a further pregnancy. And a similar small proportion of each group, 4 per cent, said they would make the same choices for a future delivery even if it meant there was a slightly increased risk to the baby's life and health.

Induction and the differences between live and still births

The basic question here is whether induction contributes to or explains any of the observed differences between those who had a still birth and those who had a live baby. To try to answer this, four groups have been compared: those induced and those not induced who had still births and who had live births.

The difference in the proportion who were given *epidurals* was confined to the induced: 18 per cent of the induced still births were given one, 9 per cent of the induced live births. This probably relates to the cause of still birth: if women are induced because the fetus is dead or known to have severe congenital malformations, the mother may be more likely to be given an epidural (numbers are too small to test this).

Anxieties during labour were most often reported by the non-induced who had a still birth: 58 per cent of them reported some anxiety compared with 29 per cent of the non-induced who had a live birth. Among the still births those who were induced were less likely to report anxieties (42 per cent compared with 58 per cent who went into labour spontaneously). Possibly the induced felt reassured that some action was being taken. But there is also some indication that the induced had a better relationship with nurses and midwives. Three-quarters of the induced among both groups described the *nurses and midwives as 'very helpful'* during their labour, while among the non-induced those who had had a still birth were less likely to do so, 63 per cent against 76 per cent of the non-induced who had had a live birth; and twice as many described them as 'not very helpful', 11 per cent against 5 per cent.

The smaller proportion of short, under six hours, first-stage labours among the still births was confined to the induced; for them the proportion was 33 per cent compared with 52 per cent of the induced live births. Possibly labours take longer to get going at an earlier stage of gestation.

Whereas a small proportion of induced live births were delivered on a *Sunday*, there was no such fall off among still births that were induced and delivered on that day of the week. This might suggest that Sunday is a relatively hazardous day to have an induction, but an alternative explanation is that Sunday inductions are more likely to be emergencies.

Similar proportions of the induced in both groups were *delivered by a doctor* but, among the non-induced, those who had a still birth were more likely to be delivered by a doctor – 42 per cent compared with 19 per cent.

So none of the observed differences in those who had still and live births were attributable to the higher induction rate for the still births, but some of the differences were confined to those who were induced and some to the non-induced.

In conclusion

A study of induced labour which was confined to women who had had a live birth only would exclude an important group, since induction was relatively common among those who had a still birth, particularly among still births associated with toxaemia and with congenital abnormalities of the nervous system.

Relatively few still births, 2 per cent, occurred among women whose pregnancy had lasted for forty-three weeks or more. So an increase in inductions among women past their expected date of delivery could do little to decrease the current still-birth rate. Nevertheless, the estimated still-birth rate among women whose pregnancy had lasted for forty-three weeks or more was greater than among those delivered at forty-one weeks.

Although the women's descriptions of their experiences during labour were in many ways similar to those of women who had a live birth, there is some indication that those who had a still birth found the nurses and midwives less helpful. But the evidence of the lack of understanding and information *after* the birth is clear-cut. Present services, possibly because of inexperience, often lack humanity in coping with this now relatively uncommon tragedy.

4 Induced and non-induced labour and delivery

In this chapter the experiences of women during labour and delivery are compared for those whose labour was induced and for those whose labour started spontaneously. Only those who had a live birth are included. Initially it was thought that it might be possible to compare those who were induced for medical reasons and those who were induced for social ones but, as was shown earlier, all but 3 per cent of those who were induced perceived some medical reason for the procedure. This means that there was presumably some additional cause for anxiety about nearly all those who were induced, and it is impossible to distinguish the differences that are due to the induction itself and those that result from the reason for the induction.

Starting labour

The process of starting labour was, of course, very different for the two groups. Most of those whose labour started spontaneously had to get to the hospital after their labour started; a few, 5 per cent, had their babies at home (O'Brien 1978), and 4 per cent had been admitted to hospital before they went into labour. More, 20 per cent, of those who were induced had been in hospital for three or more days before they were induced. Only 1 per cent of the induced had home births, and fewer of those who were induced had their babies in the place that was initially arranged, 85 per cent against 90 per cent. But there was no difference between the two groups in the proportion who were transferred from one hospital to another during labour, 2 per cent.

Those who were admitted in labour were asked when they first started having labour contractions and when they were admitted to hospital. The time between these two was then calculated. For one in eight it was less than an hour; for just over a quarter it was between one and three hours; another quarter waited between three and six hours; and a third for longer. One reason for delay was uncertainty about whether they were in labour or not.

When asked if they had any particular reason for wanting the baby to arrive at a particular time or before a particular time, 17 per cent of the women in both groups said they had. The most common reason (given by 5 per cent of all mothers) was wanting it to arrive on a family birthday or anniversary: 'On my parents' wedding anniversary. It's sentimental really.' Others wanted the time to fit in with their arrangements – either those related to the birth (3 per cent): 'My husband booked his holiday for the time it was due and couldn't change it'; or with holidays and other plans (another 3 per cent): 'I wanted him to be born during the summer holidays so that my mum could have the other boy.' A further 2 per cent were anxious to avoid a long wait: 'I hoped the baby would arrive early – when I least expected it – so I wouldn't have that awful wait beforehand'; 'I'd have liked her to arrive when she was due. It didn't worry me, only the hanging around.' Rather less than 1 per cent said they wanted the baby to arrive at a particular time in order to avoid induction: 'I wanted her not to be late as I was induced the first time and didn't want to go through that again – it was too painful.'

Similar proportions in both groups, one in twenty, would have preferred the baby to arrive a bit later than it did. A higher proportion would have preferred it to be earlier: over a third, 37 per cent, of those who had an induction, a quarter of the others. The main reasons for wanting it earlier were that the baby was overdue and the pregnancy too long; 13 per cent of all mothers made this type of comment: 'After the actual date you get a bit impatient'; 'Just hanging round those ten days was a flaming nuisance'; 'I'd have liked her to arrive on time. She was a week late. They might not have had to start me off if she'd been on time. I'd have liked to have started off myself. I don't think it would have been so painful.' Six per cent of those who were induced mentioned that an earlier arrival would have prevented that pro-cedure: 'One week earlier would have meant a more natural labour.' Five per cent of all mothers mentioned the hot weather: 'It seemed endless going over. I suppose it was the long, hot summer that did it. I would have been more comfortable not going over as I did.'

It is perhaps surprising that, as induced labours generally occurred rather later in pregnancy than spontaneous ones, and more of the mothers who had an induction wished the baby had arrived rather earlier, relatively few of them did anything to try and 'bring it on'. When asked, 'Was there anything that happened to you or that you did before you went into labour that you thought might have helped to bring it on? I don't mean anything that the doctors or nurses did after you were admitted', only 4 per cent of those who were induced compared with 23 per cent of those whose labour started spontaneously answered affirmatively. The difference may have arisen because the induced less often did things that were successful. Another possibility is that those who were induced were less energetic and therefore less likely to go into labour spontaneously, or that they were as energetic but this did not start off their labours so they did not report their activities.

Nine per cent of the non-induced mothers reported some sort of strenuous activity: 'decorating two bedrooms', 'a good walk in the woods', 'spring cleaning', 'gardening', and so on. Four per cent had taken a hot bath, or castor oil. Five per cent mentioned something a doctor or midwife had done: 'They said the internal had done it.' Two per cent thought some argument or emotional upset might have contributed: 'I put a hole in my freezer by trying to clean it, and I was so worried what I was going to tell my husband I went into labour that afternoon'; 'I was upset, I'd been smacking Stephen for something and chased down the street after him.' Other things that were mentioned by 1 per cent or less were accidents, sexual intercourse, bumpy car rides, alcohol, and a variety of things such as 'Mum kept giving me hot cups of tea' and 'I was constipated – pushed a lot on the toilet'.

Pain relief and pain

Women who were induced were more likely to have been given some pain relief during labour than those whose labours started spontaneously, 89 per cent compared with 79 per cent. Among those who were *not* given any, the proportion who said they would have liked to have been given something was a quarter, and this did not differ between the induced and the others. Twice as many of the induced as the others said they were given an epidural, and more also reported some other type of injection to relieve pain. The figures are in *Table 25.*

Table 25 Pain relief and induced and spontaneous labours

	Induced labours	Labours starting spontaneously	All labours**
	%	%	%
Pain relief*			
None	11	21	19
Epidural or spinal anaesthetic	9	4	5
Other injection	72	62	64
Something to inhale	52	52	52
Other	4	6	5
	%	%	%
First given pain relief			
At right time	70	69	69
Preferred sooner	16	16	16
Preferred later	4	5	5
Rather none at all	6	8	7
Other comment	4	2	3
	%	%	%
Given enough/too much pain relief			
Given enough	70	73	72
Liked more	7	7	7
Given too much	9	7	8
Mixed views/other comments	14	13	13
	%	%	%
Glad had what did			
Yes	73	75	74
No – rather nothing	6	7	7
No – rather something else	13	11	12
Mixed views/other comments	8	7	7
Number of labours	522	1599	2134
Number of labours for which pain relief given	463	1260	1733

* Percentages add to more than 100 as some had more than one type of pain relief.
** Excluding elective Caesarean sections but including thirteen uncertain if induced.

The proportions who said they were given pethidine were 38 per cent of the induced, 29 per cent of the others, but many mothers did not know what drug they had been given. There was no difference in the proportion who said they had something to inhale. Neither were there any differences between those who were induced and those who started labour spontaneously in the proportion who thought they were first given pain relief at the right time (just over two-thirds of those receiving pain relief), the proportion who thought they were given enough pain relief (nearly three-quarters of those who had any), and the proportion who felt glad they had what they did.

There were big variations between hospitals, particularly in the use of epidurals. In twenty-one of the thirty-seven hospitals at which at least twenty of the sample births occurred none of the sample had an epidural, but in one the proportion was two-fifths. Twenty per cent of those in 'teaching' hospitals had an epidural compared with 3 per cent of those in 'non-teaching' acute ones, and 3 per cent of those in maternity hospitals. Women having their first baby were comparatively likely to have an epidural: 9 per cent of them had one, against 3 per cent of other women.

In spite of the lack of difference between those induced and the others in their general assessment of the pain relief, there were some differences amongst those who were given epidurals. On balance the induced seemed to have derived more benefit from their epidurals. Only 4 per cent of them said it did not help at all compared with 14 per cent of those who went into labour spontaneously (a difference that did not quite reach the 5 per cent level of statistical significance). Possibly this is because an epidural can be timed more effectively when labour is induced. On the other hand, more of those who were induced and had an epidural felt they would have liked more of it: 24 per cent against 9 per cent; and, if this comparison is confined to those who thought the epidural helped a lot, the proportion who wanted more of it was 21 per cent of the induced, 2 per cent of those whose labour started spontaneously. There was no difference in their views on other types of pain relief, so all mothers have been taken together in *Table 26*.

Epidurals were most helpful and tablets least so. Those who had been given an inhalant were asked if they had any problems with it, and over a quarter, 28 per cent, reported some difficulty. Ten per cent said it had made them feel sick or dizzy or given them other physical side effects. Nine per cent had difficulties using it: 'I hadn't the strength to push it hard onto my face. If you don't push hard enough you suffocate, breathing in the rubber mask. I eventually managed and my husband helped'; 'I didn't know how to inhale it. I was taking too much. The nurse said to me hadn't I been to relaxation classes, you're taught to use it there. The nurses took it away from me.' But even those

Table 26   Views on different types of pain relief

	Epidurals	Other injection	Inhalant	Tablets
	%	%	%	%
Helped				
A lot	83	45	52	32
A little	5	33	32	33
Not at all	10	19	14	33
Other comment	2	3	2	2
	%	%	%	%
Given enough	75	77	81	74
Liked more	16	10	7	11
Given too much	7	10	10	14
Other comment	2	3	2	1
Number of mothers given that type of pain relief (= 100%)*	111	1369	1119	95

* Small numbers for whom inadequate information was obtained have been omitted when calculating percentages.

who had had lessons sometimes had problems:

> 'It didn't seem to work because the way we'd been told you start to breathe as soon as your stomach tightened up. I tended to get the pain and then the contractions so I was always too late. It was all back to front to what I'd been told.'

Three per cent said they had taken too much, and as a result: 'knocked myself out', 'got a bit drunk', 'fainted', or: 'Towards the end I couldn't feel the contractions at all, they had to tell me when they were coming. If I'd been more aware I could have been more help and maybe the whole thing could have taken less time.' Another 3 per cent said they did not like the mask over their faces – 'it frightens you'. Two per cent had problems with empty cylinders or ones that ran out. Other difficulties were: 'I tend to panic. I sort of can't push and suck gas and air at the same time. I can't relax. I panic – I rejected it'; 'It made me dopey, although the midwife had told me it didn't. When they put the mask on I said I couldn't breathe and they said, "Of course you can breathe". Then they had a look and found they hadn't turned it on at all.'

Comparisons of length of labour are difficult because the start of

Table 27   Length of first stage for induced and spontaneous labours

Length of first stage : hours	Induced labours	Labours starting sponta- neously	All labours
	%	%	%
Less than 1	2	1	1
1 but less than 2	7	4	5
2 but less than 3	9	6	7
3 but less than 6	31	21	24
6 but less than 9	20	16	17
9 but less than 12	12	13	13
12 but less than 18	8	17	15
18 but less than 24	3	8	6
24 or more	4	11	9
Could not say	4	3	3
Number of labours (= 100%)	519	1586	2118

induced labour is likely to be more clearly defined. But taking the length of time women said they had contractions during the first stage,[1] induced labours on average were shorter than ones that started spontaneously: 15 per cent of the former lasted twelve hours or more, 36 per cent of the others. The distributions are in *Table 27*.

There was no difference in their estimates of the length of the second stage, nor in the length of time the mothers said they had 'bad pains'. (Ten per cent had no bad pains, 14 per cent had them for less than half an hour, 16 per cent for between half an hour and an hour, 19 per cent for one hour but less than two, 14 per cent for two to three hours, 16 per cent for three to six hours, and 11 per cent for six hours or more.) Assessment of pain is subjective, and the fact that the length of time the women said they had bad pain is related to the proportion who were given some form of pain relief can be interpreted in different ways. The relationship is show in *Table 28*.

The proportion who were given pain relief was lowest, 54 per cent, for those who reported bad pains for a short period. After that the proportion rose with the length of time they had bad pains.

The proportion who did not have bad pain at all was highest, 26 per

[1] Mothers were asked when they first started having contractions and then when they started pushing down. The difference between the two times was then calculated.

Table 28   Bad pain and pain relief

Length of time had bad pains	No pain relief	Some pain relief	Proportion given pain relief	
	%	%		
Not at all	14	9	73%	(203)
Less than 15 mins.	14	4	54%	(117)
15 mins. but less than 30 mins.	11	7	74%	(170)
30 mins. but less than 45 mins.	11	8	75%	(172)
45 mins. but less than 1 hour	10	7	75%	(165)
1 hour but less than 2 hours	18	20	82%	(411)
2 hours but less than 3 hours	10	14	86%	(285)
3 hours but less than 4 hours	4	9	91%	(163)
4 hours but less than 6 hours	5	9	89%	(169)
6 hours or more	3	13	95%	(238)
Number of births (= 100%)	394	1699	81%	(2134)*

* Includes thirty-eight for whom inadequate information was obtained about the length of time they had bad pains.

cent, among those who had an epidural, did not differ significantly from 8 per cent among those given other types of analgesic, and was 14 per cent among those who had none. Once again the epidural seemed more effective for the induced. Thirty-five per cent of the induced who had an epidural reported no bad pains, against 18 per cent of the non-induced who had one.

The intensity of pain was assessed by using a five-inch scale, the bottom end of which was marked 'no pain' and the top end the 'worst pain can imagine'. Mothers were asked to indicate their pain at different stages on this scale, and this was subsequently classified from nil ('no pain') to six ('worst pain can imagine'). The averages for the induced and non-induced groups at different stages are shown in Table 29.

The only difference that emerged for the three main stages was for delivery: those whose labours started spontaneously rated their pain as rather greater at this stage than women whose labours were induced. But fewer of the former said they were given any, or any extra, pain relief at that stage, 22 per cent compared with 28 per cent of the induced. There was no difference between the two in the intensity of the worst pain that was reported – in spite of the high proportion among the induced who were given some form of pain relief.

Table 29   Pain score at different stages for induced and spontaneous labours

	Induced labours	Labours starting spontaneously	All labours*
Pain during first stage	3.2 (521)	3.1 (1581)	3.2 (2116)
Pain during second stage	3.3 (496)	3.5 (1534)	3.4 (2043)
Pain during delivery	2.8 (489)	3.1 (1525)	3.0 (2027)
Worst pain	4.3 (521)	4.3 (1586)	4.3 (2168)

* Includes thirteen uncertain if induced.

As a higher proportion of the induced had their membranes ruptured artificially, the average pain related to this can be assessed in two ways: first in relation to all mothers in the two groups. For them the pain score was highest among the induced, 1.3 against 0.6. But if the score is based only on those for whom the procedure was performed the scores are 1.5 for the induced, 1.8 for the others. Possibly when membranes are ruptured artificially for reasons other than induction it is done under less ideal conditions – or possibly mothers perceive it as more painful if they do not understand or accept the reasons for it.

When the source of the worst pain is considered, it was the actual delivery for a higher proportion of the spontaneous labours (37 per cent compared with 30 per cent), while for more of the induced it was artificial rupture of the membranes (9 per cent against 3 per cent); but of course this procedure was more common for the induced – 90 per cent compared with 33 per cent reported it.

Specific sorts of pain and other symptoms that mothers were asked about were feeling or being sick, headaches, backache, feeling hungry, and feeling thirsty. Feeling thirsty and having backache were the most commonly reported symptoms – by 59 per cent and 55 per cent of mothers respectively. The one which showed a significant difference between the induced and non-induced groups was being thirsty – it was more often reported by the induced, 63 per cent compared with 57 per cent of those going into labour spontaneously. This difference was not accounted for by the pain relief they were given, although those who had been given some pain relief were more likely to have felt sick (32 per cent against 22 per cent of those not given anything), to have been sick (21 per cent against 12 per cent), and to complain about being thirsty (61 per cent against 52 per cent). Having or not having an epidural did not affect the proportion who reported backache or being thirsty, but was related to sickness. The proportion who felt sick was 48 per cent of those who had an epidural, 31 per cent of those given some other type of pain relief, and 22 per cent of those not given anything, while the proportions who actually were sick were 36 per cent, 20 per cent, and 12 per cent in those three groups.

Help during labour

Three-tenths of the mothers said they had some worries and anxieties during labour. This proportion was similar for those who were induced and for those who went into labour spontaneously. Many of their anxieties were simple and almost inevitable: 'Just if he was all right. I worry at the last minute–"Is he all right?"'; 'That the child would not survive or would be damaged in some way.' Sometimes the anxieties stemmed from events or symptoms during pregnancy or even earlier: 'If he would be all right after having German measles contact and the vaccination'; 'I was thinking about my blood pressure and I kept thinking about my dad because he died at____hospital.' Long labours seemed to cause anxieties in some instances: 'I still had the fear [of actually having a baby] – and it seemed to drag on for so long'; 'I wondered why it was so long and when everything was going to happen.' More of the women whose labours lasted twenty-four hours or more reported anxieties, 44 per cent compared with 28 per cent, but within the labours lasting under twenty-four hours there was no marked trend. For others, the care they received sometimes seemed to contribute to their anxieties rather than allay them. One had been frightened because the doctor from the ante-natal clinic had come to see her while she was in labour: 'I thought something was the matter. I thought they'd fetched the doctor.'

Going to preparation classes was not related to reports of anxiety during labour, neither was the woman's parity.

Those who had found the nurses and midwives very helpful, those who said the staff had been very understanding about their pain, and those who did not have any difficulty getting in touch with a doctor or nurse were, not unnaturally, less likely to report worries and anxieties than those whose experience had been less satisfactory. This can be seen from *Table 30*.

Similar proportions of both the induced and those going into labour spontaneously described the nurses and midwives during their labour as 'very helpful', 'fairly helpful', and 'not very helpful', and similar

Table 30   Help and anxieties during labour

	Proportion reporting anxieties*		All mothers
Nurse and midwives during labour:			%
Very helpful	27%	(1629)	77
Fairly helpful	32%	(327)	15
Not very helpful	50%	(102)	5
Other comment	52%	(69)	3
Hospital staff:			%
Very understanding	25%	(1368)	65
Fairly understanding	34%	(498)	23
Not understanding	47%	(163)	8
Other comment	43%	(94)	4
Had difficulty getting in touch with doctor or nurse at some stage:			%
Yes	39%	(137)	7
No	28%	(1882)	93
All mothers	29%	(2131)	

* Excluding those having elective Caesarean sections.

proportions of the two groups thought the staff were 'very understanding'. The overall proportions are in *Table 30*.

Examples of ways in which staff were not felt to have been helpful were: 'I did [worry] when she kept saying the baby's heartbeat wasn't normal. I was anxious for it to be born and the doctor kept saying I was too anxious'; 'Right at the end when the midwife wouldn't believe she was nearly coming out and I got in a panic.' Just over half, 54 per cent, of those who had been worried had discussed their anxieties with someone, but nearly half, 46 per cent, had not done so. Some reasons for not talking about it were: 'Because they can't tell themselves until the baby is born'; 'There was too much going on at the time'; 'I was in too much pain'; 'I just sat on the bed and I was wondering – I just didn't ask. No reason really.'

Midwives or nurses were the most common confidants of those with anxieties, and just over a third of those with problems had talked to them; one in seven had discussed their anxieties with their husband; a tenth with a doctor. For the most part they found the people they talked to helpful. Sixty-one per cent described them as very helpful, 16 per cent as fairly helpful, and 19 per cent as not very helpful (the rest made other comments). More, 71 per cent, of those who had talked to their husbands described it as very helpful compared with 56 per cent of those who had talked to a doctor or nurse.

Inductions tend to be associated with 'high technology'. The drugs are often administered through an intravenous drip and machines may be used to measure contractions or to monitor the baby's heartbeats. Eighty per cent of those who were induced said they were attached to a drip and 29 per cent to a machine (these percentages include 27 per cent who were attached to both). The comparable proportions among those whose labours started spontaneously were, of course, much lower: 22 per cent had a drip, and 12 per cent were attached to a machine (including 7 per cent to both). When those who had been restricted in these ways were asked if they minded or whether they would have preferred to be able to move around more freely, nearly two-thirds in both groups said they did not mind. But this means that 30 per cent of the induced compared with 8 per cent of the others felt they would have preferred to be able to move around more. Some comments were: 'A bit uncomfortable as all the pain was in my back and it was resting on my back. But I would rather know the baby's heartbeat was all right'; 'I thought it was damn ridiculous. They kept looking at it and saying, "Ooh that was a strong pain wasn't it?". You're telling me it was a strong pain and I was writhing in agony! But for the heartbeat it's good'; 'I didn't mind the drip but I didn't like that baby heart machine. I asked him to turn the volume down. It frightens you.' Half of those attached to a machine said it was measuring their contractions, four-fifths that it was monitoring the baby's heart, 3 per cent did not know what it was for.

More of those who were induced said the baby's heart had been checked while they were in labour, 92 per cent compared with 80 per cent of those starting spontaneously, and more of the induced said it had been checked by a machine, 32 per cent against 17 per cent, whereas similar proportions in each group said it had been checked by a stethoscope (9 per cent) or by a 'trumpet' (57 per cent). (Some said it was checked in more than one way.)

Given these rather different levels of activity, it was perhaps surprising that similar proportions of women in both groups, slightly less than half, said they had been left alone at some stage. But fewer of the induced had apparently minded being left alone: 27 per cent of the induced who had been left alone at some stage said they would rather someone had been there, 35 per cent of the others. Possibly the induced were left for shorter periods, and certainly on average their labours were not so long. And more of the induced said they *felt* they could get in touch with a doctor or nurse at any time if they wanted one, 95 per cent compared with 87 per cent. But there was no difference in the proportion who said they had had any difficulty in getting in touch with a doctor or nurse when they needed one – 7 per cent of mothers said this had happened. Some descriptions of what happened were: 'After my husband went I was on my own and I got a bit panicky. They were a long time coming when I rang, and I have my babies quickly'; 'Only one was on duty. She kept disappearing. She was busy'; 'I had to shout, because I couldn't reach the bell with me being on the drip.'

> 'I didn't know there was a bell there at the time. The baby started coming before I went into the delivery room. I could feel the baby coming down. I shouted for someone and they didn't hear me. I shouted again – a cleaner or someone fetched Sister. It was my fault really for not pressing the bell, but I didn't know it was there.'

When asked who or what had been the greatest help during the first stages of their labour, rather more of those who had spontaneous labour said no-one or nothing, 17 per cent compared with 11 per cent of the induced. More of the induced said a nurse or midwife had helped them most, 43 per cent against 36 per cent, but fewer of the induced said that preparation classes had helped them most, 2 per cent compared with 4 per cent. (There was no difference in the proportions who said they had been to preparation classes: a third of both groups.) Possibly the content of some preparation classes is less relevant to induced than to spontaneous labour. Their husband was the next most commonly mentioned person, after a midwife or nurse, as helping them most. Three-tenths of both groups said this, and, when only those whose husband was there at some stage are considered, this proportion rises to two-fifths; when their husband was present at all more women found him, rather than the nurses, their greatest help. This was so for both induced and spontaneous labours.

Husband's role

The event that marks a woman's transition to motherhood also marks a man's to fatherhood. But the man's role in this transitional event is inevitably less, and may be insignificant.

The husband was rather more likely to have been there at some stage during labour if it was induced, 72 per cent, than if it started spontaneously, 67 per cent. This presumably is because it is a planned procedure generally starting during the day and therefore easier to make arrangements. But the proportion of *births* at which the husband was present (a third) did not differ; neither did the proportion of labours (a quarter) for which the husband was there all the time vary. Half of the women whose husbands had not been there all the time would have liked him to be there or there for longer. Rather fewer, 38 per cent, of the husbands in this situation were thought by their wives to have wanted to be there. Once again these proportions were similar in the two groups.

The great majority of both the women and their husbands had appreciated it when the husband had been present[2] – and the more stages they were present at the higher the proportion who were reported to be glad about the experience. (The proportion of mothers who were glad he had been there increased from 88 per cent of those whose husbands had been there at only the first stage to 99 per cent when he had been present at all stages. And the proportion of wives reporting that their husbands had been glad to be with them increased from 85 per cent to 98 per cent.)

Husbands were much more likely to have been present at some stage when it was the first baby, 82 per cent, falling to 64 per cent of those having their second, 56 per cent of those having their third, and less than half of those having a fourth or later one. Many of the husbands with other children are likely to have been involved in looking after or making arrangements for the other members of the family. And, of course, labour was longer for first births than for later ones: 41 per cent of women having their first baby had contractions for twelve hours or longer, 24 per cent of other mothers. The proportion present at the actual birth also fell, but much less steeply, from 39 per cent of first births, 37 per cent of second, 31 per cent of third, and 23 per cent of fourth and later ones. So if the number who were present at the birth is expressed as a proportion of those present at some stage, this is rather lower for first births than for others, 48 per cent compared with 56 per

[2] (If husband there at all.) 'So were you glad he was there or would you rather he'd not been there – or not there at certain stages?' 'So do you think he was glad to be with you?'

cent. This seemed to be because forceps were more often used for first births.

Whether or not husbands were present also varied with social class. Just over three-quarters, 77 per cent, of middle-class fathers were there at some stage compared with two-thirds of those in skilled manual occupations and less than half, 45 per cent, of those in unskilled jobs, while the proportion present at the birth declined from 54 per cent of those in social class I to 16 per cent of those in social class V. Men in white-collar jobs may find it easier to get time off work and to make arrangements for the care of their other children. Among those women whose husbands were not present all the time, similar proportions of middle- and working-class women would have liked him to be there or there for longer. But of the women whose husbands were there at some stage, rather more of the middle- than of the working-class women said they were glad about it, 97 per cent against 93 per cent, and slightly more middle- than working-class husbands appreciated the experience, 95 per cent against 92 per cent. Although these last two differences are statistically significant, the most important point is that over nine-tenths of both middle- and working-class wives and husbands were glad of the opportunity to be together during the woman's labour and delivery, but that working-class couples were less able to arrange it. This difference is similar to the one found by Earthrowl and Stacey (1977) in their study of children in hospital: there were few class differences in attitudes but major variations in availability of resources and some differences in their treatment by hospital staff.

An indication that middle-class couples may have been more aggressive in demanding to be together comes from their response when the women who would have liked their husbands to be there or there for more of the time were asked if they thought the hospital would have agreed to this : 31 per cent of the middle class compared with 18 per cent of the working class said no. It seems probable that one reason for more of the middle-class husbands being there was that more had asked about it or just assumed it was possible. And this meant that if the hospital did not encourage or allow this, more of the middle class were aware of this policy.

Some comments about husbands not being allowed in were: 'Husbands have to go to classes about childbirth before they're allowed to stay. We didn't realize this beforehand. My husband has delivered babies when he was an ambulanceman but it made no difference'; 'I don't think they do with your first one at___hospital. I think they do with your second and third'; 'I don't think so. Another girl wanted her husband in but they wouldn't let them stay. Nurse at clinic said if they could avoid it they didn't want father there because the rooms were small.' One mother whose husband was present most of the time but who would have liked him there all the time explained:

> 'I was very lucky in the event, because the one Sister who doesn't allow men in the labour ward went off duty. They told me she wouldn't allow it and I told her it was my baby and I wanted my husband there and he would be there. She said, "We'll see". I was glad the way it happened because I know my husband would have got his way whatever. He was determined to be there.'

Several women said their husbands had not been allowed to stay because they had a forceps delivery: 'Apparently they don't allow them in for a forceps birth – but they didn't tell him that. They just said he'd have to go out for a few minutes, and by the time he came back it had been born.'

The assisted delivery rate[3] was relatively high when husbands had been present at the first stage only, 26 per cent, or at the first and second stage but not the birth, 54 per cent. It was low, 4 per cent, when husbands were present at the birth, but also seemed comparatively low when husbands were not there at any stage, 8 per cent, compared with 18 per cent among those whose husbands were there at some stage. This last difference was partly accounted for by variations in parity and in length of labour, but when these were held constant there were still some significant differences. Among those whose labour lasted twelve hours or more, the assisted delivery rate for those having their first baby was 18 per cent if the husband was not there, 37 per cent if he was, and the corresponding proportions among those having a second baby were 0 per cent and 13 per cent. Possibly husbands agitate for something to be done – or possibly forceps are occasionally used as a reason for asking the husband to leave? This might contribute to the slightly higher assisted delivery rate among the middle class (17 per cent) compared with the working class (13 per cent).

Among the thirty-seven hospitals with twenty or more deliveries in the sample, the proportion at which the husband was present at some stage varied from 20 per cent to 95 per cent.

[3] 'Were any instruments used to help the baby out?'

Delivery

The proportion delivered by Caesarean section was 3 per cent of those whose labour started spontaneously, 4 per cent of those who were induced – a difference that could well occur by chance. And the length of time they had been in labour before they had a Caesarean was also similar: just under a quarter of each group had been in labour for twenty-four hours or more. Three per cent of both groups had breech deliveries but the proportion of deliveries that were assisted was higher among the induced, 21 per cent, than the spontaneous labours, 13 per cent. The difference persisted when those who had epidurals were excluded, the proportions then being 18 per cent of the induced and 12 per cent of those starting labour spontaneously. Among those who had an epidural the proportion of assisted deliveries was 56 per cent. Overall the proportion was 15 per cent.

Reasons for the use of instruments were perceived rather differently by women who were induced and by those who went into labour spontaneously. More of those who were induced said instruments were used because the baby 'wouldn't come', was 'lodged', or 'too high up' (of those with an assisted delivery, 20 per cent of the induced against 11 per cent of those going into spontaneous labour gave this as the reason), while more of those whose labour started spontaneously said that the reason for using instruments was that the mother was too tired to unable to push for some reason (26 per cent against 20 per cent). But these differences might have occurred by chance.

Induced births were more likely to be delivered by a doctor (27 per cent compared with 17 per cent), but this seemed to be mainly because of the high proportion of assisted births among the induced. If the comparison is confined to births at which no instruments were used, the proportion said to have been delivered by a doctor was 10 per cent of the induced, 7 per cent of the others – a difference which might occur by chance.

The proportion who had episiotomies[4] was higher among the induced than the non-induced, and the difference in the proportion among those having a vaginal delivery who had to be stitched was in a similar direction. Among those who did not have episiotomies the proportions who were stitched were similar in the two groups. The figures are in *Table 31*. The difference in the proportion having episiotomies disappeared when comparisons were made between those

---

[4] 'Did they cut you at all?'

Table 31   Induction, episiotomies, and stitching

	Induced		Spontaneous start		All mothers	
Proportion with episiotomies	54%	(498)	48%	(1541)	49%	(2052)
Proportion stitched	74%	(500)	69%	(1544)	71%	(2057)
Proportion stitched among those *not* having episiotomies	41%	(219)	40%	(773)	40%	(1001)

The figures in brackets are the numbers on which the percentages are based (= 100%).

having or not having an assisted delivery.

The pain score associated with the insertion of the stitches was similar for the two groups, but more of the women who had been induced said the stitches caused them a lot of pain and discomfort afterwards: 40 per cent against 34 per cent of those starting labour spontaneously. Again this seemed to be because more of those who were induced had assisted deliveries; if this is held constant there is no significant difference between the two groups.

Summing up

It is clear from many of the comments made by mothers that they found a pregnancy that went on after their expected date of delivery tedious, frustrating, and uncomfortable. At this stage a number of them deliberately engaged in activities which they hoped would encourage the onset of labour. Some felt they had been successful. So induction might be seen as a more reliable and sophisticated, as well as medically sanctioned, way of doing what they might otherwise try to do themselves. For those induced because they were overdue, the procedure might well be welcomed as a means of cutting short a trying period and bringing forward a welcome event.

Induction has other advantages for the mother, in that it is easier to arrange for husbands to be present and to carry out other procedures such as giving epidurals at an appropriate stage.

But there are disadvantages. In spite of a higher rate of pain relief among the induced, levels of pain during labour were similar among those who were induced and among those whose labour started spontaneously, suggesting that induced labour is intrinsically more painful. Induced labour may be shorter on average, but as measured by the length of time mothers felt they had bad pains induction has no advantage. Many women found the mechanics of induction restricting and induced labours more often resulted in an assisted delivery.

In an attempt to get an overall assessment of how women felt about their labour, they were asked: 'Looking back now, do you consider your labour was a pleasurable experience, rather unpleasant but endurable, or a nightmare?' Replies are shown in *Table 32*.

Table 32   Views on labour

	Induced	*Spontaneous start*	*All mothers**
	%	%	%
A pleasurable experience	31	35	34
Unpleasant but endurable	52	48	49
A nightmare	10	9	9
Other comment	7	8	8
Number of mothers (= 100%)	497	1543	2053

* Excluding those who had an emergency or an elective Caesarean section but including thirteen uncertain if induced.

If anything, those who were induced were slightly less likely to say it had been a pleasurable experience—but the difference might have occurred by chance (.05 < p < .10).

In fact, this assessment seemed a relatively insensitive index. Although rather more of those who had not been left alone at any stage regarded their labour as a pleasurable experience (38 per cent compared with 29 per cent of those who had been left alone), this proportion did not vary with parity or with the husband's presence at some stage during labour. However, other data show that the husband's presence was greatly appreciated when it was arranged. This was true for both middle- and working-class couples but, for one reason or another, opportunities were greater for the middle class. When husbands were present they generally gave much help and support. More opportunities and encouragement for them to be there is an obvious recommendation from this study.

5 Mother and baby

This chapter looks at the first few months of the babies' lives, and the data from this survey about the relationship between the mothers and babies during this time. It starts by describing the first contacts between mothers and babies, then goes on to consider their experiences while they were in hospital and later when they returned home. Once again a major concern is the comparison of induced and non-induced labours.

First contacts

'I was thrilled to ribbons that he was there and that it was over and that it was a boy.'

'Glad because she was a girl and it was over. I was very sleepy.'

'Like a dream sensation. Feel like you're in a fantasy world. A mixture of joy and relief.'

'Very difficult to describe – sort of a good feeling. You don't think about the pain, you just think how good it is.'

'Pleased – is it all right? Then I felt proud that I was a mum. I didn't think much at the time – just so long as she was O.K.'

These were some of the descriptions the mothers gave of their feelings at the time the baby was born. Ecstasy and relief were not the only reactions: 'Exhausted'; 'I burst into tears. I was thrilled because it was a girl – just delighted. Very, very drowsy because of the pethidine – kept nodding off. It just took effect as soon as she was born'; 'I was in a lot of pain. I was concerned about the pain in my hand [from the drip] and I wanted that taken out more than anything.'

Rather more mothers who had been induced said something was done to the baby to start him or her breathing: 26 per cent compared with 20 per cent.[1] The *British Births Survey 1970* found that the proportion of babies taking more than three minutes until the onset of regular respiration was much greater, 5.1 per cent, for the induced group than for the non-induced, 3.3 per cent, but point out, 'this could however reflect the risk inherent in the reason for induction rather than that of the induction itself' (Chamberlain *et al.* 1975:104).

Only a minority, 36 per cent, of the mothers said they held their baby straightaway – before the afterbirth was delivered. This proportion was similar for those who were induced and for those whose labour started spontaneously. Most (94 per cent) of the comments from those who had done so were enthusiastic: 'I thought he was lovely. Thrilled – that was the best bit'; 'Lovely – it was beautiful. I couldn't believe she looked so fat. She was so aware'; 'I was really pleased. They let my husband hold her as well.' But the experience was not always entirely idyllic: 'I just about got my hands on him then I was sick'; 'It was very difficult because of my hand [still attached to the drip] so I gave him back.'

Many of those (three-fifths) who had not held the baby straightaway said they did not mind: 'I didn't mind. I could see him, which was enough at that point. They were checking him over'; 'Not bothered. It's wicked really, but if it had been a girl I might have felt differently. He wasn't offered to me. It was only an initial reaction. By the time he'd been taken away, dressed, and brought back the feeling had disappeared'; 'They showed her to me and then took her away. I didn't really mind.' Some included in this group would have liked to hold the baby but accepted the hospital procedure:

'I would have loved to have held him for that second – but they took him away to wash him. I understood that they had to take him away to wash him, I wasn't upset – I just accepted it really. I was so relieved it was all over, I wasn't seriously bothered about not holding him.'

One in seven of those who had not held their babies said they were

[1] 'Did they do anything after the baby was born to help him/her to start breathing?'

too tired: 'I didn't mind. I was so tired and worn out. I certainly did not feel that so-called urge of maternal instinct that one reads about'; 'I wasn't in any condition to hold her. I think I would have dropped her.' A slightly higher proportion, 16 per cent, had been upset and disappointed: 'I would have loved to have touched her while she was all bloody and messy.'

Most of those who held the baby at this stage said they did so for as long as they wanted (four-fifths). A few, less than one in fifty, felt they were left holding the baby too long, almost a fifth said the baby was taken away too soon.

The most frequent reason why mothers said they did not hold the baby straightaway or were not able to hold the baby for as long as they wanted to was that the baby or the mother was being cleaned or washed first. Just over a third said this. A quarter gave reasons related to the afterbirth. Nearly a fifth, 17 per cent, said the baby needed resuscitation or some special care such as being in an incubator. One in eight said they themselves were too tired or shaky, one in twelve that they had to be stitched first, and a small group, one in seventeen, that their husband had held the baby first.

Just over half, 52 per cent, of the mothers who did not hold their babies straightaway were able to do so within twenty minutes. For a tenth the delay was between twenty minutes and an hour, and for one in twenty it was between one and three hours. A third did not hold their baby for three hours or more after it was born, including one in ten for whom the interval was twenty-four hours or longer. Many of the long delays were related to the baby going into a special care unit, but others were less easily explained. Two comments from mothers who had not held their babies until twelve hours or more after they were born were: 'I asked to have him and I was told that babies weren't washed until they were twelve hours old and I couldn't have him until then'; 'I don't know [the reason for delay]. I was all right and so was the baby. I would have liked to have held him straightaway, but I didn't ask. They were very busy.'

Small babies, weighing less than $5\frac{1}{2}$ lb, were less likely to have been held straightway (20 per cent compared with 36 per cent of babies weighing $5\frac{1}{2}$ lb or more), but there was no consistent trend with weight among the heavier babies. If instruments had been used in the delivery or if the mother needed to be stitched, this also made it less likely that the baby would be held straightaway (the proportions were 23 per cent of the assisted deliveries, 39 per cent others; 34 per cent of the 'stitched', 42 per cent of the others). The proportion varied more widely between the twenty-four study areas from 19 per cent to 53 per cent – the highest proportion being in Newcastle. Between thirty-seven hospitals with twenty or more vaginal deliveries in the sample, it varied from 9 per cent to 62 per cent.

Care in the first few days

Most of the births, 96 per cent, were in hospital, so early contacts between mothers and babies were in an institutional setting. The length of time mothers spent in hospital after the birth is shown in *Table 33*, together with their feelings about their length of stay.[2]

Table 33   Length of stay in hospital after birth and mothers' views about this

| Length of stay: days | All mothers having baby in hospital | Mothers' views on length of stay | | | | Number of mothers* (= 100%) |
		Rather leave earlier	About right	Rather stay longer	Other comment	
	%					
Less than 2	6	15%	74%	10%	1%	136
2 but less than 3	19	13%	70%	16%	1%	391
3 but less than 4	5	32%	55%	12%	1%	97
4 but less than 5	4	29%	64%	6%	1%	93
5 but less than 6	8	32%	58%	10%	—	168
6 but less than 7	9	32%	62%	5%	1%	181
7 but less than 8	11	32%	64%	4%	—	223
8 but less than 9	11	39%	56%	4%	1%	227
9 but less than 10	8	38%	58%	4%	—	168
10 or more	19	43%	53%	3%	1%	392
All mothers having hospital births	2084	31%	61%	7%	1%	2076

* Eight mothers did not give us their views about their length of stay.

A quarter of the mothers spent less than three days in hospital after their baby was born. They were the ones most likely to regard their length of stay as 'about right', the others being fairly evenly divided between those who would have preferred a shorter or longer stay. At the other end of the scale, a fifth stayed in hospital for ten days or more and, while just over half of them felt that had been 'about right', over two-fifths would have preferred to come out earlier:

'I should think five or six days would be enough. By then I'd learnt all I needed to know and the rest of it was a waste of time. I didn't get

[2] 'How long after the birth did you stay in hospital?' 'Would you have preferred to come out earlier or to stay longer, or do you think it was about right?'

any rest in hospital. In one way it was boring, but you couldn't just lie in bed. You seemed to be hanging about waiting to bath the baby and waiting for meals.'   (In hospital nine days after birth.)

There was no difference in length of stay between those having an induced or a spontaneous onset to their labour, so the need for an induction did not apparently relate to the length of need for care after delivery. There were wide variations in the twenty-four study areas. The proportion who spent less than two days in hospital ranged from none to 37 per cent, while the proportion in ten days or more varied between 2 per cent and 36 per cent (at one hospital this last proportion was 55 per cent).

Mothers having their first baby stayed in rather longer on average than those having a second or later one (7.9 days compared with 5.5 days), but there was no clear trend among the higher parities.

There was a slight tendency for mothers of lighter babies to stay in hospital rather a longer time than mothers of heavier ones, but the relationship between birth weight and length of stay was not strong. (The correlation coefficient was -0.12).

'Induced' babies were slightly heavier on average than those born after labour started spontaneously, 7 lb 7 oz against 7 lb 5 oz. But, when length of pregnancy was held constant, there was no significant difference between the induced and the others.

Among the hospital births, 5 per cent of the babies were with their mothers all the time during the first two days, and nearly half were with their mothers during the day. These two proportions were similar for the induced and for the others, but more of the induced, 26 per cent against 21 per cent of the others, spent time in a nursery or special care unit. However, the majority, four-fifths, of both groups of mothers said that they saw as much of their baby during that time as they wanted to, 17 per cent felt they saw him or her too little, and 3 per cent would rather he or she had not been with them so much.

When mothers were asked whether their babies cried a lot, an average amount, or a little at night and during the day, there were no differences between the two groups – but their sleeping patterns were assessed slightly differently. After an induced labour, babies were more often said by the mothers to have slept 'very well' during the day (69 per cent compared with 62 per cent), and 'not well at night' (11 per cent against 7 per cent). It may be that induction sometimes leads to different sleep patterns and rhythms.

When mothers were asked if the baby had any particular problems early on, such as jaundice, being premature, or any abnormalities, more of the induced (31 per cent) than of those arriving after a spontaneous labour (25 per cent) were said to have had jaundice. There were no differences between the induced and the others in the other problems. Eight per cent of the babies were said to be premature, 9 per cent to have some abnormality, and 7 per cent had other problems. One per cent had died after birth.

As expected, the mothers themselves more often said they had problems or complications because of high blood pressure after the birth if they had been induced than if their labours started spontaneously (4 per cent compared with 1 per cent), and more of the induced reported various obstetric problems (apart from bleeding, which was reported by 4 per cent in the two groups) – 12 per cent against 7 per cent. Similar proportions reported problems with lack of sleep, 2 per cent, and nerves, depression, or anxiety, 3 per cent. Over half in each group said they had felt weepy at some stage while they were in hospital or in the first few days after the baby was born.

Two-fifths said they had slept 'very well' while they were in hospital, three-tenths 'fairly well', and three-tenths 'not well'. These proportions were similar for the two groups, as were the proportions, 78 per cent, who said they were offered or given sleeping pills: 6 per cent who had asked for them and 64 per cent who had taken them. Forty-four per cent said they had been 'very comfortable' while they were in hospital, 38 per cent 'fairly comfortable', and 17 per cent 'uncomfortable'. (One per cent made other comments.) The proportion who were uncomfortable was higher among the induced, 23 per cent, than among those whose labours started spontaneously, 15 per cent, but this was partly because more of the induced had an assisted delivery. However, even among those who did not have an assisted delivery, the proportion who said they had been uncomfortable was 19 per cent of the induced, 12 per cent of those whose labour started spontaneously.

Feeding

Half of the mothers said they had had no discussion before the baby was born about feeding the baby: a quarter had been asked simply whether they wanted to breast or bottle feed, and the others had had some discussion about breast feeding (8 per cent) or bottle feeding (1 per cent) or both (19 per cent). Three-fifths of those who had discussed breast feeding said that the people they had discussed it with had suggested they should do something in preparation. As might be expected, these proportions were similar for women who were induced and for those whose labours started spontaneously, but feeding was more often discussed with women having their first baby: two-thirds of them had some discussion compared with just over two-fifths of other mothers.

Just over half the mothers, 53 per cent, said they had intended to breast feed their babies; 45 per cent did not intend to do so, and 2 per cent were uncertain.[3] Half had tried to do so – 88 per cent of those who had intended to breast feed, 4 per cent of those who had not intended to do so, and 32 per cent of those who had not made up their minds beforehand.

Thirteen per cent of those who had intended to breast feed but did not, and 57 per cent of those who had not intended to do so but did, said they had been influenced by professionals to change their plans.

Some comments by those who had been persuaded to try breast feeding were: 'I didn't know anything about breast feeding and the Sister said why didn't I try so I did, and I'm really pleased I managed it'; 'I bottle fed him in hospital. Nobody had shown me how to breast feed Lyn [last baby] so I decided to bottle feed this time. When I got home the midwife said, "Why not try breast feeding?" So I did and I'm glad'; 'When I got home I was full of milk and the nurse who came said, "Why don't you try", so I did and it worked. It's so much easier and cheaper. It was a relief to me.'

But they were not all success stories: 'The nurse tried to persuade me when I went in, so I did to keep them quiet, but I only did it at home for three days, then I went to the doctor.'

'I wasn't going to breast feed but they bullied me into it at hospital. They said it was much safer, cleaner, better for baby and you. Since they tried so hard I thought I'd have a go. It was all right in hospital because I was resting, but once I got home it was too tiring – much easier to give her a bottle.'

Some comments from those who had been dissuaded from breast feeding were:

'The doctor said milk is very watery with Caesareans – the doctor at

[3] 'And before you had the baby did you think you would try to breast feed him/her at first or not?'

the hospital said that the first time. Then the nurse asked why wasn't
I [breast] feeding, and I told her and she said it was a load of old
balls. I probably could have done it this time – there was so much
milk it was dropping off me.'

'The doctor looked back at my chart and saw that I'd only breast fed
the last one five days so he advised me not to. He said I could if I
wanted to but he advised not. So I thought I would start as I meant
to go on.'

Women who were induced were no more or less likely to breast feed
their babies than women whose labours started spontaneously and, if
the comparison is confined to babies born in hospital,[4] they fed them
for similar lengths of time.

The length of time mothers had breast fed their babies is shown in
Table 34 for all mothers and for those of different parities. Breast
feeding was more common for first babies than for later ones. A
comparatively high proportion of those having their first baby gave up
in the first week (17 per cent compared with 9 per cent for later births
of those who had breast fed at all).

Table 34 Breast feeding and parity

How long breast fed entirely	Pregnancy order				All mothers
	First	Second	Third	Fourth or later	
	%	%	%	%	%
Not at all*	36	56	63	66	50*
Less than a week	11	4	3	5	7
A week but less than a month	11	9	8	9	10
One month but less than two months	10	8	10	5	8
Two months or more but not still breast feeding	8	7	6	2	7
Still breast feeding	16	13	8	8	13
Partially only	8	3	2	5	5
Number of mothers (= 100%)	799	830	312	165	2108

* Includes 1 per cent who tried to breast feed but did not do so.

[4] Babies born at home were more likely to be breast fed and to be breast fed for
longer than those born in hospital (O'Brien 1978).

Table 35 Breast feeding and social class

How long breast fed entirely	Social class						
	I Profes-sional	II Inter-mediate	III Skilled Non-manual	Manual	IV Semi-skilled	V Un-skilled	Unclas-sified
	%	%	%	%	%	%	%
Not at all	27	38	46	57	62	67	45
Less than a week	9	5	8	6	7	6	7
A week but less than a month	12	12	10	9	9	9	7
One month but less than two months	10	12	8	9	6	2	7
Two months or more but not still breast feeding	8	9	11	5	4	4	13
Still breast feeding	32	19	13	9	7	8	14
Partially only	2	5	4	5	5	4	7
Number of mothers *(= 100%)*	194	359	236	821	296	110	90

Breast feeding was also strongly related to social class (see *Table 35*). Women married to men in non-manual occupations were not only more likely to try breast feeding their babies, but when they did so they were more likely to do so for longer. A third of the breast-feeding middle-class women were still breast feeding their baby at the time of interview, compared with a fifth of the working-class women.

Breast feeding related not only to characteristics of the mothers but also to their experiences and perceptions of hospital policy and the helpfulness of staff. The proportion who breast fed at some stage varied from 24 per cent to 92 per cent among the thirty-seven hospitals where twenty or more of the women in the sample had their babies.

Mothers were more likely to breast feed their babies if this had been discussed with them beforehand – and even more likely to do so if given some advice about preparation beforehand. This can be seen from *Table 36*, which also shows that mothers were more likely to breast feed if they found the nurses helpful about it and if they thought the nurses favoured breast feeding. But if they started to breast feed, none of these factors was related to the time they went on doing so. Altogether 53 per cent of the mothers found the nurses 'very helpful' about feeding, 27 per cent found them 'fairly helpful', and 13 per cent

Table 36   Breast feeding in hospital and mothers' experiences

	Proportion breast feeding at all	Number of mothers (= 100%)
Preparation:		
Feeding not discussed	39%	1000
Asked which wanted to do	47%	458
Method(s) discussed but no preparation	54% ⎱ 73%	199
Given advice about preparation for breast feeding	86% ⎰	293
Nurses thought to:		
Favour breast feeding	59%	1076
Favour bottle feeding	52%	65
Encourage whichever wanted	42%	488
Not to bother	24%	336
Nurses found to be:		
Very helpful about feeding	57%	1037
Fairly helpful	42%	537
Unhelpful	35%	263
Able to feed baby:		
Whenever wanted	71%	380
Fixed times only	43%	1509

'unhelpful' (7 per cent made other comments).[5] Doctors were much less likely to be seen as helpful: 90 per cent of the mothers said the doctors gave them no help with this.

Another factor related to breast feeding was whether they were able to feed their baby whenever they wanted or could only do it at fixed times. Only a fifth of mothers in hospital said they were able to feed their babies whenever they wanted to, while three-quarters said they could only do so at fixed times. (The rest gave other answers.) Many more of those in the former group had breast fed their babies. It may be that hospitals were more permissive about this when mothers were breast feeding, and more rigid about bottle-feeding schedules, but this cannot be the complete explanation, since 67 per cent of those who

[5] 'How would you describe the help the nurses gave you over feeding the baby? Were they very helpful, fairly helpful, or unhelpful?'

were breast feeding could only do so at fixed times, and 11 per cent of those who bottle fed entirely could do so whenever they wanted. Within the twenty-four study areas, the proportion who said they could feed their baby whenever they wanted varied from 4 per cent to 48 per cent – the highest proportion being in Newcastle.

Permissiveness about feeding times also related to the length of time mothers went on breast feeding. Seventeen per cent of those who started breast feeding gave it up within a week if they were only able to do so at fixed times, compared with 6 per cent of those able to feed their baby whenever they wanted to.

One women who was breast feeding and would have preferred a more flexible approach said: 'Although she was a good baby it worked out she wanted to be fed every three hours and then sleep all night, so she spent a lot of time crying with hunger. They can't read the clock.' But most seemed to accept the system and adapt to it: 'If everyone did that it would be organized chaos. You have to wake them up to feed them'; 'It seemed a shame to have to wake them up and shake them about – but I can see that they have to have a routine.' However, when mothers could feed their babies whenever they wanted, more of them preferred it that way, 95 per cent, than if they could do so only at fixed times, 55 per cent. These proportions were similar for those who breast fed and for those who did not.

Back home

Mothers were asked whether they felt very confident, fairly confident, or not very confident about looking after the baby when they first got home – or when they were left to look after their baby alone if the baby was born at home. Not surprisingly, their replies were strongly related to their experience, as is shown in *Table 37*.

Did any of their experiences during pregnancy and labour relate to their feelings of confidence about looking after their baby? There was no indication that having an induction or, when parity was held constant, holding the baby straightaway affected women's confidence in looking after their babies. Nor, apparently, did going to baby-care classes increase their confidence. Just over a quarter, 28 per cent of those having their first baby in hospital said they had been to such classes while they were in hospital, and a further 5 per cent said there were such classes but they had not been to them. Over half, 59 per cent, of those who had been, described them as 'very helpful', 33 per cent as

Table 37   Mothers' confidence and parity

| Mother felt: | Number of previous pregnancies (ending in a live or still birth) | | | | | All mothers |
	None	One	Two	Three	Four or more	
	%	%	%	%	%	%
Very confident	17	49	58	65	75	40
Fairly confident	52	43	33	28	16	43
Not very confident	30	7	9	4	7	16
Other comment	1	1	—	3	2	1
Number of mothers *(= 100%)*	805	850	320	127	44	2149

'fairly helpful', and 8 per cent as 'not very helpful'. But two-thirds of those having their first baby said there had not been any classes for them to attend while they were in hospital, and just over half, 53 per cent, of this group, or a third of all those having their first baby, said they would have liked to go to such classes. Among those having a second or later baby, 27 per cent said such classes were available, 19 per cent had been to them, and one in six would have liked to go to such classes but there were not any available.

The proportion who had been to classes was relatively low, 11 per cent, among those who were in hospital for three days or less, rose to 16 per cent for those in for four days, and to 26 per cent for those who were in longer. But the proportion of those having their babies at home who were given advice or instruction about caring for the baby by the midwife was much higher, 54 per cent. In addition, 69 per cent of those given advice or instruction by the midwife after a home birth found it very helpful compared with the 53 per cent who described the hospital classes in those terms. So people who have a short stay in hospital would probably benefit from a home visit from the midwife. Certainly those who had such a visit seemed to appreciate it more if their stay in hospital had been relatively short. Overall, 70 per cent described their contacts with the midwife since they left hospital as 'very helpful', and this proportion was 78 per cent of those who were in hospital for less than four days, 68 per cent of those who were in hospital for four to seven days, and 59 per cent of those who were in for longer. Three per cent of all mothers and 11 per cent of those who had not seen a midwife

Table 38   Help at home and parity

Sources of mothers' help	Mother's parity					All mothers
	None	One	Two	Three	Four or more	
	%	%	%	%	%	%
Husband	89	90	87	90	87	89
Mother	50	52	45	37	30	49
Mother-in-law	27	25	25	16	15	25
Sister or sister-in-law	26	27	30	30	34	27
Other relatives	11	9	13	21	28	12
Friends or neighbours	25	38	48	44	49	35
Local authority home help	—	1	—	3	2	1
Private home help	—	2	2	7	—	2
Other source	5	4	3	3	2	4
No-one	3	2	2	2	2	2
Number of mothers (= 100%)	817	860	326	126	47	2179

since they got home said they would have liked one to call and see them.

Women's various sources of help when they first got home (or, for those having their baby at home, at first after the baby was born) are shown in *Table 38*.[6] Husbands were most commonly mentioned, then mothers, and then friends or neighbours. Mothers and mothers-in-law were less likely to help as family size increased, while friends and neighbours were more likely to do so, presumably because they often helped by looking after older children, or because neighbours know each other better when they have children.

Whether or not they had a local authority home help was unrelated to social class, but the proportion who had a private home help declined from 6 per cent among those married to men in professional and intermediate occupations to 1 per cent among others. Working-class women were no more or less likely than middle-class women to get help from their mother or mother-in-law, but more of the working class said their sister or sister-in-law had helped them: this proportion rose

---

[6] 'When you first got home did you have any help from: your husband, your mother, your mother-in-law, sister or sister-in-law, any other relatives, friends or neighbours, a local authority home help, a private home help, anyone else?'

from 16 per cent in social class I to 45 per cent in social class V. This may be a reflection of different family sizes.

Middle-class husbands were more likely than working-class ones to take time off as holidays, while working-class ones more often than middle-class ones took unpaid time off. But even among the working class, taking holiday time was the most common way in which husbands freed themselves to help (see *Table 39*).

Seventeen per cent of the mothers said they would have liked more help: 7 per cent wanted help with housework or cooking or shopping, 6 per cent help with looking after the baby, 2 per cent help with older children, and 2 per cent general help or 'help with everything'. Over a quarter, 27 per cent, of those whose husbands had not helped at all said they would have liked more help.

Earlier, in the chapter on still births, the people whom mothers had talked to about having the baby and looking after the baby were described. Husbands, friends or neighbours, and their own mothers were the ones most frequently mentioned, and these three and health visitors were the ones most commonly described as the most helpful. One in ten mothers said they would have liked to talk to someone else about this sort of thing, and half of this group said they would have liked to talk to a nurse, health visitor, or midwife; a third would have preferred a doctor, one in ten a relative, and one in twelve a friend.

Twenty-nine per cent of the mothers said they had some problems when they first got home (or 'at first' for home births), and two-fifths of this group wanted more help.

Other subjects the mothers were asked about related to the baby's health, the baby's sleeping habits, and their own health. For none of these were there any major differences between the induced and the others but, as will be shown, there were two small differences related to the mothers' own health.

The proportion reporting some problems with the baby after they got home decreased from 82 per cent of those having their first to 58 per cent of those having their fourth pregnancy, but rose somewhat to 66 per cent of those having a fifth or later one. The most common problems were feeding or wind, reported by 50 per cent of all mothers, crying by 36 per cent, and sleeping at night by 31 per cent. Around the time of interview, when most of the babies were three or four months old, the proportion reporting problems had dropped from 75 per cent to 42 per cent. By that stage one in eight were still having problems with the baby sleeping at night. The average number of nights the

Table 39 Social class variations in when husbands helped

When husband helped	Social class							All couples
	I Profes-sional	II Inter-mediate	III Skilled Non-manual	Manual	IV Semi-skilled	V Unskilled	Unclas-sified	
	%	%	%	%	%	%	%	%
Before or after work only	20	21	17	23	23	17	17	21
Took holiday	51	51	64	48	41	28	46	49
Took time without pay	2	3	3	7	8	11	6	6
Given time off	8	4	2	2	4	3	10	3
Unemployed	1	1	1	3	4	20	4	3
Other	10	8	5	6	9	5	2	7
Did not help	8	12	8	11	11	16	15	11
Number of couples (=100%)	196	365	238	842	311	114	94	2162

baby awakened the mother or father in the seven days before the interview was 1.6. This did not differ between those who were induced and the others, but varied from 57 per cent who did not wake them on any night to 13 per cent who woke them on all seven. The longest length of time the baby was said to have slept during this period was generally between ten and fourteen hours (62 per cent had slept that long); 8 per cent slept longer, but 4 per cent had not slept for as long as six hours at a stretch. Again, this was unrelated to induction.

When the baby needed to be picked up at night, over half, 56 per cent, of the mothers always did this themselves. A fifth of them *usually* did it, a fifth shared it on an equal basis with their husbands, and in one family in twenty the father did it more frequently than the mother. These proportions were similar for babies who were always bottle fed and did not differ between middle- and working-class couples.

When asked to rate their own health since they got home[7] as very good, fairly good, or not good, half the mothers said it was very good, two-fifths said fairly good, and one in ten not good. Slightly more of those who were induced said it was not good, 12 per cent compared with 8 per cent of those whose labour started spontaneously – but of course this may be related to the reason for the induction. The various symptoms they reported[8] are shown in *Table 40*. Irritability, undue tiredness, and nerves or depression were the most common ones.

Piles, discharge, infections, and being 'turned off my husband sexually' were some of the other symptoms more commonly reported.

Painful intercourse was much more often reported by those who had had their first baby than by others (25 per cent against 9 per cent). This may be because of the increased use of forceps or because of more frequent intercourse among younger mothers (Cartwright 1976). Constipation was less often reported by the higher parity mothers, while backache was reported more often (31 per cent of mothers having their first baby reported constipation, against 21 per cent of those having their fourth or later pregnancy, while the comparable proportions reporting backache were 18 per cent and 28 per cent). There was no variation with parity in the frequency with which other symptoms were reported.

The one symptom that showed a difference between those whose

---

[7] Those who had a home birth were asked about their health since ten days after the birth.

[8] 'Have you had any of these symptoms or problems: Trouble with your breasts, bleeding, trouble passing water, constipation, nerves on depression, irritability, backache, undue tiredness, painful intercourse, anything else?'

Table 40   Symptoms or problems reported
by mothers since they got home*

	%
Trouble with breasts	20
Bleeding	15
Trouble passing water	5
Constipation	28
Nerves or depression	45
Irritability	52
Backache	30
Undue tiredness	46
Painful intercourse	15
Anything else	20
None of these	13
Number of mothers (= 100%)	2179

* Or in the ten days after the birth for those having
their babies at home.

labour was induced and those whose labour started spontaneously was
nerves or depression: this was reported by 48 per cent of the former
compared with 43 per cent of those whose labour started
spontaneously – not a large difference, but one not too likely to occur
by chance (.02 < p < .05). Unfortunately we have no measure of the
duration or intensity of the symptoms. More of the working- than of
the middle-class women reported nerves or depression (48 per cent
compared with 40 per cent), the proportion rising from 34 per cent in
social class I to 51 per cent in social class V. There were no clear social
class trends or differences in the other symptoms that were reported.
The difference between middle- and working-class women in the
reporting of nerves and depression is similar to differences in the
prevalence of psychiatric disturbance found in another study (Brown,
Bhrolchain, and Harris 1975).

Women who reported nerves or depression were no more or less
likely to have seen a midwife, health visitor, or general practitioner
since they returned home, and there was no association with their
length of stay in hospital; but those who were nervous or depressed
were less likely to regard their baby as 'very easy' to look after and
more likely to regard him or her as 'rather difficult'.[9] This can be seen
from Table 41.

[9] 'On balance would you describe [your baby] as: a very easy baby to look
after, a fairly easy baby to look after, a rather difficult baby to look after?'

Table 41   Mothers' nerves and views of their babies

	Mothers reporting nerves or depression	Mothers who did not report nerves or depression	All mothers
	%	%	%
Baby described as:			
Very easy to look after	57	68	63
Fairly easy	34	27	30
Rather difficult	8	4	6
Other comment	1	1	1
Number of mothers			
(= 100%)	955	1194	2149

Table 42   Mothers' experiences of labour and views of their babies

	Labour considered to be		
	A pleasurable experience	Rather unpleasant but endurable	A nightmare
	%	%	%
Baby described as:			
Very easy to look after	71	61	56
Fairly easy	24	32	34
Rather difficult	4	6	10
Other comment	1	1	—
Number of mothers			
(= 100%)	693	981	192

This is a classic chicken and egg situation. It is obviously impossible to know which way round the association goes: a difficult baby may lead to a nervous or depressed mother while a mother who is nervous or depressed may communicate her unease to the baby or may be more inclined to perceive the baby as difficult.

Mothers' assessments of their baby as easy or difficult to look after were not related to whether their labour was induced or started spontaneously. Nor did the assessments vary with their parity or social class. Breast-fed babies were more often described as very easy, the proportion falling from 73 per cent of those who were breast fed for two months or more to 66 per cent of those breast fed for two to four weeks, 60 per cent of those breast fed for less than two weeks, and 59 per cent of those who were not breast fed at all.

A relatively high proportion of mothers who had found their labour a pleasurable experience found their babies very easy to look after. This can be see from *Table 42*. But here too interpretation is difficult. It may be that for women with a cheerful and optimistic temperament labour is more likely to seem pleasurable and babies easy to look after.

Post-natal care

All but 8 per cent of mothers said they had taken their baby to a 'well-baby clinic' – or to a general practitioner for a check-up when the baby was well. The average number of times they took the baby was 4.9. This was much higher for first babies, as can be seen from *Table 43,* which also shows that women were more likely to go for a post-natal examination after their first baby than subsequently.

There was no indication that mothers who were meant to have their post-natal examination done by a general practitioner were any more or less likely to attend than those who were meant to have it at a hospital. This was so overall and when parity was held constant.

Attendance at baby clinics did not vary with social class, but the proportion of mothers who had had their post-natal was 95 per cent of middle-class mothers, compared with 89 per cent of those married to men in skilled manual occupations, 86 per cent of those married to men in partly-skilled ones, and down to 74 per cent of those married to men

Table 43   Clinic and post-natal attendance and number of previous pregnancies

Number of previous pregnancies	Average number of times baby taken to clinic	Proportion of mothers who had had postnatal examination	Number of mothers (= 100%)
None	6.0	94%	817
One	4.3	92%	861
Two	4.5	85%	327
Three	3.0	74%	127
Four or more	3.3	68%	47

Table 44 Social class, parity, and attendance at post-natal examination

| Social class | Proportion who had not had post-natal | | | | All mothers |
| | Number of previous pregnancies | | | | |
	None	One	Two	Three or more	
I Professional	4% (80)	5% (74)	9% (35) ⎫		5% (195)
II Intermediate	2% (141)	4% (158)	10% (42) ⎬ 21% (43)		6% (368)
III Skilled { Non-manual	4% (100)	1% (104)	12% (26) ⎭		3% (239)
III Skilled { Manual	6% (305)	10% (337)	13% (139)	35% (72)	11% (855)
IV Semi-skilled	7% (122)	10% (108)	26% (46) ⎫		14% (312)
V Unskilled	36% (33)	21% (38)	26% (27) ⎬ 26% (50)		26% (114)
Unclassified	3% (36)	10% (39)	* (10)	* (8)	8% (92)

* Inadequate numbers.

in unskilled jobs. This difference persisted when parity was held constant – see *Table 44*, which shows the proportion who had *not* had a post-natal examination. The trend is very similar to that found in an earlier study (Cartwright 1970:199).

All except 4 per cent of the mothers said they had seen a health visitor since the baby was born. The majority, 60 per cent, had found her 'very helpful', 26 per cent described her as 'fairly helpful', and 14 per cent as 'not very helpful'. Their views of her helpfulness were unrelated to their number of previous pregnancies. There was no difference between middle- and working-class mothers in their assessments of the health visitor's helpfulness, but within the working class those in social class V more often described the health visitor as very helpful, 68 per cent compared with 59 per cent of other working-class mothers.

Most mothers, 91 per cent, had seen a general practitioner since the birth of their baby, but this proportion was comparatively low, 76 per cent, for those having their fourth or later babies. Just under half the mothers, 48 per cent, said the general practitioner had been to see them at home, and this varied in the opposite direction: relatively few mothers having their first baby had had a home visit from the general pratitioner, 41 per cent against 53 per cent of other mothers. At the same time rather more middle-class than working-class women had been visited at home by a general practitioner: 52 per cent compared with 46 per cent.[10] A fifth of those who had not seen a general practitioner and a quarter of those who had not seen a health visitor would have appreciated a visit from them.

Summing up

The differences following an induced rather than a spontaneous labour were relatively few in number and small in size. But all the ones that did exist indicated that mothers and babies were less healthy and happy when labour was induced. Some of the differences may be related to the initial cause of the induction but, as the proportions reporting nerves or depression during *pregnancy* were similar for the two groups, this seems an unlikely explanation for the more frequent reporting of nerves and depression among women whose labour was induced. This finding seems to merit further investigation.

The more important findings in this chapter relate to the prevalence rates of two restrictive practices. Nearly two-thirds of the women were not able to hold their baby as soon as he or she was born, although the overwhelming majority of those who were able to do so were enthusiastic about it. In addition just over three-quarters of the mothers said they were not able to feed their babies in hospital when they wanted to, but could only do so at fixed times. Data from the study suggest that a flexible and permissive approach was appreciated by mothers, encouraged them to try breast feeding, and enabled more of those who tried to establish breast feeding. It may be that a less rigid regime demands more resources. In terms of hospital maternity services overall it would seem that more resources might be freed for this by reducing the average length of stay in certain areas and hospitals. Nearly a third of the mothers would have preferred a shorter stay in hospital and the proportion whose length of stay was ten days or more after the birth varied greatly between study areas.

The proportions of mothers holding their babies immediately after birth, breast feeding them, and being able to feed them whenever they wanted to also varied widely in ways that indicated clear differences in policy between hospitals.

Already, in the first few months of their lives, some class variations emerged in the treatment of babies. The most notable one, also found in other studies (Martin 1978) was in breast feeding. There were no class differences in the frequency with which babies were taken to clinics, but rather more middle-class women had had a home visit from

[10] An analysis of home and surgery consultations by age and social class in one general practice revealed proportionally more home visits for patients in social class I than for those in other social classes at all ages (Jarman, unpublished).

their general practitioner, although working-class mothers more often reported nerves or depression. So as well as differences in the home environment there were differential services, and it is likely that general practitioners would know more about the environment of the babies from middle-class homes in the same way as they know more about their elderly patients when these are middle class than when they are working class (Cartwright and O'Brien 1976).

6 Mothers' information, views, and choices

Up to now, the main emphasis in this report has been on mothers' experiences, although their views on certain aspects of these experiences have also been considered. This chapter is concerned with the information mothers were given at different stages of their childbearing, with the sources of this information, with mothers' desire for further information, with their views on induction and their preferences for different types of care in the future, and with their perceptions about the choices they had for different types of care during their recent childbearing experience.

Discussion and sources of information before birth

Once people have experienced an event it is often difficult for them to recall how they felt about it beforehand and what their knowledge and expectations were before it happened. Inevitably their experience colours their perceptions of the past. Nevertheless, mothers were asked: 'Disregarding what you know now and looking back to the time before you went into labour (this last time) – *at that time* did you feel you knew enough about what to expect or did you feel you would like to know more, or did you feel you would rather not know what to expect?' Replies are shown in *Table 45* for women having their first baby and for others.

A fifth of the women having their first baby had felt they would like to know more, and another fifth did not know what to expect but felt they would rather not know. After the event the proportions making

Table 45 Adequacy of knowledge beforehand for women having their first baby and others

	Women having first baby	Women having second or later births
	%	%
Knew enough	62	82
Like to know more	18	10
Rather not know	19	7
Other comment	1	1
Number of mothers (= 100%)	816	1358

these sorts of assessments increased slightly – a quarter of those having their first baby said that looking back now there was something they wished they had been told or warned about before they went into labour, and another quarter did not feel this but said that was not because they realized what it would be like but because they thought it was better not to know (see *Table 46*).

The things they most often wished they had been warned or told about beforehand were induction (3 per cent of all women and 10 per cent of those who were induced), the analgesic or anaesthetic (2 per cent), the pain (2 per cent), and untoward events (2 per cent). One mother described how she had felt about induction in these terms:

'I'd have liked to have been warned about what could possibly

Table 46 Mothers' retrospective assessment of their knowledge

	Mothers having first baby	Mothers having second or later babies
	%	%
Something they wished they had been warned or told about beforehand	24	13
Realized what it would be like	49	76
Better not to know	23	10
Other comment	4	1
Number of mothers (= 100%)	803	1327

occur if the baby was overdue – and the causes. That was awful. No-one explained. They all just came and did what they had to – no explanations whatsoever, and left me. I realized he [the baby] was late but I was not prepared about induced labour at all at any of the lectures. I wish I had been prepared in some way because it was so frightening. I was scared stiff having things done and not knowing what it was, as though you were just a thing – not a person with a mind.'

Another put it more succinctly: 'They should explain what they are going to do when they start mucking about.'

Those who were having their first baby were asked where they got most of their ideas from about what the actual process would be like. Books were the most frequently mentioned source, by 55 per cent, then classes, by 49 per cent, and discussion, by 45 per cent. Films and television were each mentioned by one in ten of the mothers, radio by 1 per cent. When questioned about whom they had discussed it with, three-quarters, 77 per cent, of the women mentioned their husbands, over half, 56 per cent, their friends, rather under half, 45 per cent, their mothers, and two-fifths, 42 per cent, other relatives. Discussions with professionals were mentioned less often: a quarter had talked to a nurse or midwife about it, a fifth to a general practitioner, one in ten to a doctor at hospital, and one in twelve to a health visitor. Asked to identify who or what was most helpful, 28 per cent said classes, 18 per cent books. Discussions with their mother, their husband, other relatives, friends or neighbours, and a nurse or midwife were each mentioned by between 6 per cent and 9 per cent, other sources by less than one woman in twenty.

Two-thirds of those having their first baby had been to preparation classes for childbirth, and 42 per cent of those who had done so said the classes had been their most helpful source of information. Those who had been to classes were more likely to have felt they knew enough beforehand, 72 per cent compared with 40 per cent of those who had not been to any classes; and they were less likely to say they would rather not know, 14 per cent against 30 per cent. Of those who had not been to any classes, the majority, 85 per cent, of those having their first baby said there were such classes, but 5 per cent said there had not been any, and the remainder were uncertain. So a quarter had not been to classes that were available, while 2 per cent would have liked to go to classes but did not know of any.

Table 47 Social class and sources of ideas about what the actual process would be like before having first baby

	Social class							All mothers
	I Professional	II Intermediate	III Skilled Non-manual	III Skilled Manual	IV Semi-skilled	V Un-skilled	Unclassified	
	%	%	%	%	%	%	%	%
Where got most ideas from:								
Discussion with people	33	45	46	45	50	66	28	45
Books	70	60	55	53	48	31	56	55
Classes	63	67	54	46	35	9	42	49
Films	11	14	8	11	9	9	8	11
T.V.	13	9	11	9	14	3	14	10
Radio	1	3	1	—	—	—	—	1
Other	6	9	6	6	7	9	11	7
Nowhere	—	—	—	3	5	3	3	2
	%	%	%	%	%	%	%	%
Discussed with:								
Mother	36	43	53	51	34	42	39	45
Husband	83	85	68	76	77	67	78	77
Other relatives	28	35	37	46	50	70	28	42
Friends	59	62	54	55	56	45	56	56
General practitioner	35	23	24	18	24	15	22	22
Doctor at hospital	11	16	16	9	11	—	11	11
Nurse or midwife	31	39	26	23	21	6	25	26
Health visitor	11	12	12	4	9	—	6	8
Anyone else	5	4	2	2	1	—	—	2
No-one	4	2	8	6	6	3	6	5
Number of mothers having first baby (= 100%)	80	141	100	307	121	33	36	818

Only 13 per cent of those having a second or later baby had been to preparation classes, but among those who did go the proportions who found the classes very helpful were similar, two-thirds, in the two groups; a quarter described them as fairly helpful, one in fourteen as 'not very helpful'.

Attendance at preparation classes was strongly related to social class. Among those having their first baby the proportion going to preparation classes fell from 85 per cent in social class I to 21 per cent in social class V. But among those who had not gone, the reasons they gave were similar for middle- and working-class women except that middle-class women more often said they had not had time to go (38 per cent compared with 22 per cent). A fifth gave reasons associated with the clinic, mostly the difficulties of getting there or the awkward times: 'Because they were at night and I'd have had to go into——and I couldn't make it, really.'

Working-class women were not only less likely to go to preparation classes, they also were less likely to get their ideas about the process of having a baby from books. They relied more on discussion with relatives, and were considerably less likely to have talked to a professional person about it. The data are in *Table 47*.

As their sources of information were fewer and less professional, it is not surprising that working-class mothers were less likely to have felt they knew enough before they had the baby and more likely to say they would rather have known more. The figures are in *Table 48* for mothers having their first babies. There is an increase in the minority group who said they would rather not know what to expect, from 8 per cent in social class I to 22 per cent in social class V.

A quarter of the mothers said they had had some discussion during their pregnancy with a doctor, nurse, or midwife about pain relief during labour.[1] Again this type of exchange was more common for middle- than for working-class women: the proportion who had discussed it fell from 40 per cent in social class I to 11 per cent in social class V. But this social class variation did not arise just because women in the higher social classes were more likely to ask about it. The proportion of mothers who had initiated a discussion about pain relief themselves declined from 10 per cent in social class I to 3 per cent in social class V, while the proportion who said a discussion was initiated by a professional fell from 28 per cent to 9 per cent.

[1] 'At any stage of your pregnancy did you have any discussion with a doctor, nurse, or midwife about epidurals – that is, a spinal anaesthetic, or about any sort of pain relief during labour?'

Table 48 Social class and adequacy of knowledge beforehand for mothers having their first baby

	Social class					
	I Profes- sional	II Inter- mediate	III Skilled		IV Semi- skilled	V Un- skilled
			Non- manual	Manual		
	%	%	%	%	%	%
Knew enough	81	74	63	55	52	44
Like to know more	11	14	17	20	21	34
Rather not know	8	11	16	23	25	22
Other comment	—	1	4	2	2	—
Number of mothers *(= 100%)*	80	141	100	305	122	32

Table 49 Social class and discussion of induction during pregnancy

Social class	Proportion who had discussed induction during pregnancy					
	Induced		Spontaneous labour		All mothers*	
I Professional	73%	(40)	46%	(146)	50%	(195)
II Intermediate	47%	(77)	38%	(283)	40%	(369)
III Skilled { Non-manual	66%	(50)	41%	(187)	46%	(240)
III Skilled { Manual	55%	(223)	29%	(609)	35%	(857)
IV Semi-skilled	} 57%	(97)	23%	(202)	33%	(312)
V Unskilled		(14)	17%	(100)	22%	(115)
Unclassified	71%	(21)	34%	(71)	43%	(94)
All mothers	57%	(522)	32%	(1598)	38%	(2182)

* Including those who had an elective Caesarean section.

Induction was more likely to be discussed than pain relief: 38 per cent of the women said it had been discussed,[2] and this proportion was 57 per cent of those who were subsequently induced, 32 per cent of the others. (It was only 19 per cent among those having an elective Caesarean section.) The trends with social class are shown in *Table 49* for those who were induced and for those who were not.

Those who said they had not discussed induction with any professional during their pregnancy were asked if they would have liked to talk about it with someone: 18 per cent of them said they would have liked to do so, and this proportion was 35 per cent among those who were induced. So, of all those who were induced, 57 per cent had discussed it with someone beforehand, 15 per cent had not done so and wished it had been possible to do so, while 28 per cent had not done so but were apparently quite happy about that.

Desire for further information

Towards the end of the interview, mothers were asked to review the information they were given in retrospect, and to say whether they would have liked more information about any of the things listed in *Table 50* or if they would have liked information about them earlier. Replies are shown separately for those who were induced and for others.

Two-fifths of those who were induced said they would have liked more information about induction, and this was higher than the proportion wanting more information about any other aspect of care. Altogether four-fifths of the mothers wanted more information about some aspect of their care. Other aspects mentioned by three-tenths or more of the mothers were the baby's progress before labour, during labour, around delivery, and in the first two days, and drying up the milk. A quarter had wanted more information about pain relief and about machines and gadgets that had been used.

On average, mothers wanted more information about 4.4 topics, and if anything this was slightly higher for those who were induced, 4.7, than for those whose labour started spontaneously, 4.3. An analysis by social class in *Table 51* shows that the number of topics they wanted more information about increased quite substantially and

---

[2] 'At any stage of your pregnancy did you have any discussion with a doctor, nurse, or midwife about induction – that is, starting the labour before it happens on its own?'

Table 50 Topics about which mothers wanted more information

	Proportion wanting more information			The one they would rather have been told about most		
	Induced	Sponta-neous labour	All mothers	Induced	Sponta-neous labour	All mothers
	%	%	%	%	%	%
Starting labour	21	16	17	1	3	2
Process of labour	15	13	14	1	1	1
Caesarean opera-tions	19	19	19	2	3	3
Induction	41	21	26	13	3	6
Epidural or spinal anaesthetic	26	27	26	4	4	4
Other forms of pain relief	26	26	26	4	3	3
The pushing or se-cond stage	15	17	16	2	2	2
Actual delivery	13	14	13	2	2	2
Being cut	19	19	19	—	1	1
Being stitched	19	18	19	1	1	1
The afterbirth	16	18	17	1	2	2
The machines and gadgets they use	31	27	28	6	3	4
The baby's pro-gress:						
before labour	34	32	32	3	5	4
during labour	35	33	33	6	7	7
around delivery	33	32	32	3	4	4
in first two days	32	32	32	8	6	6
later on in hos-pital	18	22	21	2	2	2
Breast feeding the baby	16	17	16	5	7	6
Bottle feeding the baby	16	14	14	1	2	2
Looking after the baby	17	17	17	4	4	4
Own progress after baby was born	23	22	22	3	3	3
Drying up the milk	31	30	30	6	7	7
Getting rid of the stitches	14	14	14	1	2	2
Anything else	8	5	6	4	2	3
Nothing	17	21	19	17	21	19
Number of mothers (= 100%)	521	1597	2178	507	1544	2109

Table 51   Social class and desire for more information

Social class	Average number of items would have liked more information about	Number of mothers (= 100%)
I Professional	3.3	195
II Intermediate	3.9	369
III Skilled Non-manual	4.4	239
III Skilled Manual	4.7	856
IV Semi-skilled	4.6	311
V Unskilled	5.5	114
Unclassified	4.1	94
All mothers	4.4	2178

with a clear trend from 3.3 in social class I to 5.5 in social class V. So the relative lack of information and discussion in the lower social classes is mirrored by a greater feeling of deprivation and desire for more information.

Desire for more information on different topics decreased with increasing parity from an average of 5.2 topics for those having their first baby to 4.1 for those having their second, 3.7 for those having their third, 3.4 for fourths, and 2.9 for fifth or later ones.

In retrospect, 50 per cent of those who were induced and with whom induction had not been discussed beforehand said they would have liked more information, or earlier information, about induction, compared with 34 per cent of those who said they had talked about it beforehand with a doctor, nurse, or midwife. So prior discussion helped to reduce feelings about inadequate communication, but was by no means always successful in doing so.

Inadequate communications seemed to contribute to the mothers' overall assessments of their experiences during labour. The average number of topics they wanted more information about was 3.9 for those who described it as 'a pleasurable experience', 4.6 for those who found it 'rather unpleasant but endurable', and 5.7 who thought it a 'nightmare'. It may be that those who had a difficult labour wanted more explanation about complications or things that went wrong. But if this is the reason for the relationship, it seems that inadequate explanations are given when difficulties arise. Alternatively, it may be that withholding information creates a nightmarish situation.

Some of the mothers had not attempted to ask or find out about the things they wanted to know about. One, who had wanted more information about pain relief, said:

'They should tell you about all the things – needles and things, so you have a choice. You never got asked about this or told nothing.' ['Did you ask anyone about this?'] 'I don't think it's my place to ask all these things. You should be approached first.'

Another woman having her first baby wanted to know more about the actual birth: 'I didn't know nothing about it – just the whole lot. I didn't think to ask anybody.' Attempts to elicit information were sometimes abortive: 'I asked and they'd come and tell you something but they were so busy they couldn't stop and explain' (wanted more information about breast feeding); 'I did ask what was happening but the question was ignored and passed off – you know the sort of thing.'

On other occasions the information that was obtained was felt to be inadequate; a mother whose baby was put in an intensive care unit for two days after a breech delivery and had not seen him for eighteen hours after the birth, nor been able to hold him until forty-three hours later, said:

'It all seemed to be like a secret, not that they did withhold anything but that's how I felt. They'd just say, "Your baby is doing fine and will probably be coming over tomorrow". When they took me just to see him in a wheelchair I was just there two minutes, looking through a window. It wouldn't have been so bad if I could have seen the nurse feeding him – sort of seeing him doing something instead of just lying there.' (She had wanted more information about the baby's progress in the first two days.)

When babies were put in intensive care units, mothers were more likely to feel they had been given inadequate information: 43 per cent of them compared with 31 per cent of other mothers had wanted more information about the baby's progress in the first two days, and 31 per cent against 20 per cent more information about the baby's progress later on in hospital. Sometimes information seemed to be withheld in a way which, to the mothers, appeared punitive:

'Most of us were in a lot of pain if bottle feeding, and the nurses were not interested and made you feel more depressed than ever. We wanted to know how to get rid of the milk and they said, "It's your own fault, you should breast feed like all mothers should". I had to wait until I got home and got tablets from the chemist.'

Views on induction and preferences for the future

Mothers were asked how they had felt about induction before they had the survey baby.[3] Again it would have been difficult for them to recollect their feelings at an earlier point in time, and almost inevitable that their recollections would be, to some extent, coloured by subsequent events. A fifth of the mothers had no views, a third had mixed feelings, another third were against it, and one in ten in favour. Those who had views were asked why they felt like that and what their views were based on.[4] A third of all the women said their views were based on other women's experiences, another third that they were based on a television or radio programme, a fifth had some personal experience, and another fifth said their views were based on something they had read. One in ten gave other answers, and some mentioned more than one source. *Table 52* shows that those with personal experience were most likely to be in favour; but even among them three were against it for every two in favour.

Among those whose views were based on television or radio programmes, the ratio of those against to those in favour was ten to one. These women will have been pregnant at the time of the Horizon programme *A Time to be Born*. Nearly half of all the groups had mixed feelings, and among those with views based on other women's experiences or on things they had read, those against greatly outnumbered those in favour.

Two per cent of women said they tried to arrange to have an induction, 6 per cent had tried to arrange *not* to have one.[5] Most of those who had tried to arrange it had asked their doctor or hinted about it: 'I didn't exactly ask but I sort of suggested to the doctor – could I go in early?'; 'The second time I saw the doctor at the hospital, late on in

[3] 'Before you had the baby did you have any feelings about induction? What?' 'So in general were you in favour of it, against it, or did you have mixed feelings or no views?'
[4] 'Is that based on personal experience, other women's experience, T.V. or radio programmes, something you've read, or what?'
[5] 'Did you do anything to try and arrange that you would or would not have an induction?'

Table 52   Views on induction before they had the survey baby and sources of those views

	Sources of views				
	Personal experience	Other women's experiences	T.V. or radio programme	Something they had read	Other
	%	%	%	%	%
In favour	21	9	5	7	16
Against	33	45	50	49	43
Mixed feelings	45	45	45	44	40
Other comment	1	1	—	—	1
Number of mothers with views (= 100%)	496	728	694	481	269

pregnancy, I told him I was in favour of being induced and he said he'd see to it.' But not all had found their doctor so compliant: 'In the last month when I'd gone over my time I tried to push for one but everyone thought she was a 7½ pounder really. I just asked if it wouldn't be better, but they were adamant they were going to wait.'

Some of those who had tried to avoid an induction had done things to start off their labour themselves: 'I took control and went on a three mile hike and it worked.' Others had tried to reduce symptoms which might have led to an induction: 'I took it easy so my blood pressure didn't go up.' One said she had delayed going into hospital until labour was properly established: 'I didn't go to hospital until I was properly in labour. I waited until my waters broke and I had a show before going in. I thought if I went in too early they'd put me on a drip like they did my friend.' Some had been quite determined about it: 'I just wouldn't sign a form – a form you had to sign for Caesareans and induction. I wouldn't have had it done no matter what they said'; 'I told the doctor they'd have to wait until the baby was ready and if they gave me an injection I would just pull it out!' Those who had tried to arrange to have one seemed to have met with rather more success: 51 per cent of them were induced, twice as many as in the rest of the sample, whereas 21 per cent of those who had tried to avoid it were induced – a proportion very similar to the rest of the sample.

The mothers' views on induction before they had the survey baby

Table 53   Reported views on induction before they had the survey baby

	Induced	Labour started spontaneously	All mothers
	%	%	%
In favour	21	7	10
Against	19	38	33
Mixed feelings	38	34	35
No views	21	20	21
Other comment	1	1	1
Number of mothers *(= 100%)*	520	1591	2173

are compared in *Table 53* for those who were induced and for those whose labour started spontaneously.

The proportions with no views and with mixed feelings were similar in the two groups. However, the attitudes of the two groups among those who held definite views differed markedly. Those who were induced were roughly evenly divided between those against and those in favour; those whose labour started spontaneously were over 5:1 against it. Possible explanations of this difference are:

1 Doctors and nurses more often discussed induction with women who were likely to be induced and as a result of these discussions women viewed induction more favourably.
2 Women's experience of induction coloured their description of their feelings in the past, and in general the experience made them less antagonistic towards induction.
3 Women who think they are likely to be induced adapt to that by becoming more favourable to induction.
4 Doctors are less likely to induce women who are antagonistic towards induction.

It is possible that all four of these processes operated to some extent. More of those who had discussed induction with a doctor or nurse were in favour of induction than those who had not had any discussion. This held both for those who were induced and for those who were not. But, among those who were not induced, the proportion against induction was also higher among those who had discussed it with a doctor or

Table 54   Discussion of induction and views on induction

	Induced		Labour started spontaneously	
	Some discussion	No discussion	Some discussion	No discussion
	%	%	%	%
In favour	26	14	9	5
Against	21	18	43	36
Mixed feelings	39	37	39	31
No views	14	30	8	27
Other comment	—	1	1	1
Number of mothers *(= 100%)*	297	223	513	1079
Ratio In favour: against	1 : 0.8	1 : 1.2	1 : 4.7	1 : 6.5

nurse: discussion did not so much affect the ratio of those who were in favour or against induction, but decreased the proportion who had no views. This can be seen from *Table 54*.

Their current views on induction were assessed by asking about their preferences if they were going to have another baby.

'I'd like to ask you a few questions about what you'd like to happen if you were going to have another baby and there were no medical complications . . . If the doctor said that shortly before the baby was due if you liked you could come into hospital on a particular day and he would put you on a drip that would start your labour and mean that the baby would arrive more quickly – would you like him to do this or not?'

Eight per cent said they would prefer an induction. This proportion was 17 per cent of those who had had an induction for the survey baby and 5 per cent of those who were not induced.

Although the proportion who would prefer to have an induction was higher among those with recent experience of one, the main finding is that a large majority of those who had had an induction, 78 per cent, would prefer not to have another one if they had another baby. This is in striking contrast to their views on having the next baby at home or hospital. The great majority, over four-fifths, would prefer to have

Table 55   Proportion preferring various types of care if they had another baby

| | For survey birth | | | | | |
| | Induction | | Epidural | | Place of birth | |
	Induced	Not induced	Had epidural	Did not have epidural	Home birth	Hospital birth
	%	%	%	%	%	%
Prefer same as last time	17	93	63	82	91	83
Prefer not same as last time	78	5	34	13	9	15
Other comment	5	2	3	5	—	2
Number of mothers (= 100%)	522	1593	110	2053	97	2083

another baby in the same type of place as they had the last one. This proportion was greater among those who had had their baby at home than among those having it in hospital (see *Table 55*). There was less enthusiasm for epidural analgesia than for home or hospital births, but nearly two-thirds of those who had had an epidural would prefer to do so again compared with less than a fifth of those who had had an induced birth.

The main reason for not wanting an induction was epitomized in this comment: 'I'd like the baby to come naturally. I wouldn't like it to be rushed if it doesn't need to be.'

Many of those who wanted an induction stressed the advantages of having a definite date: 'When you have other children it does help to make definite arrangements – everyone feels more secure. It has its disadvantages but I do think I would'; 'You can plan for someone to look after the children and everything. Having had so many false starts – you get yourself all packed up and it stops. You build yourself up mentally and then it stops'; 'Your main fear when you're pregnant is that you're going to start in a public place, so when you know you're going to be induced it takes that fear off you.'

Other reasons for wanting an induction were: 'I don't like being pregnant and I don't like walking round like a lump'; 'Towards the end you get that fed up you just want to get it over with'; 'It's so much quicker – over and done with. It's more pain but with it all over in three hours the pain is worth it'; 'I'd prefer it because presumably the baby would be smaller.'

Comparisons with previous pregnancy and labour

Women who had been pregnant before were asked to compare their study pregnancy and childbirth with the one before.

When one of the births was at home and the other in hospital, 76 per cent preferred it at home and 15 per cent in hospital, the rest saying they had no preference.[6]

Most aspects of their experience during labour and delivery were more often felt to have been better this time. One exception to this was pain. If anything, more women felt their pain this time had been worse. It may well be that memories of pain become dulled and there is a tendency to view the more recent pain as more intense. The pregnancy itself was also quite often seen as more difficult this time, but there was no clear trend with parity. As expected, a high proportion, two-thirds, of those who had recently had their second baby said their labour this time was shorter. The other indicator which was appreciably better this time for women having their second baby was their overall assessment of their experience. But, apart from these, the variations with parity, shown in *Table 56*, were not great.

Rather more of those having their second pregnancy said they were induced last time, 35 per cent compared with 25 per cent of those having a third or later one. Possibly in the past induction was more likely to be done for first births. Altogether, 31 per cent said they were induced last time, but the questioning was not so detailed as for the current birth, so it would be dangerous to conclude from this that induction rates were falling. Women who had an induced labour last time were more likely to have one this time, 35 per cent compared with 18 per cent. Moreover, this did not seem to be simply a reflection of hospital policy. Among those who had their babies in the same hospital as last time, the proportion induced this time was 37 per cent of those induced last time, 17 per cent of the others; among those who had their babies at home or in a different hospital, the comparable proportions were 33 per cent and 18 per cent.

Comparisons of induced and spontaneous labours this time and last

[6] 'Where did you have the baby the time before?' 'So that was the same as this time/different?' *If different*, 'Which did you prefer?'

Table 56 Parity and comparisons with previous pregnancies

	Number of previous pregnancies				All mothers with previous pregnancies
	One	Two	Three	Four or more	
	%	%	%	%	%
Pregnancy this time:					
Easier	24	28	28	28	25
More difficult	29	31	24	23	29
About the same	39	34	42	47	39
Other comment	8	7	6	2	7
	%	%	%	%	%
Length of labour this time:					
Shorter	68	47	43	34	59
Longer	15	31	29	36	21
Same	15	19	28	21	18
Other comment	2	3	—	9	2
	%	%	%	%	%
Pain this time:					
Better	34	30	28	28	32
Worse	38	33	28	24	35
Same	26	35	44	44	31
Other comment	2	2	—	4	2
	%	%	%	%	%
Way looked after this time:					
Better	35	32	22	30	33
Worse	11	14	10	9	12
Same	52	52	67	61	54
Other comment	2	2	1	—	1
	%	%	%	%	%
Experience – altogether:					
This time better	52	36	35	37	46
This time worse	18	23	19	24	19
Same	28	39	45	39	33
Other comment	2	2	1	—	2
	%	%	%	%	%
This baby:					
More easy	49	47	41	40	48
More difficult	22	20	20	30	21
Same	28	33	39	30	30
Other comment	1	—	—	—	1
Number of mothers (= 100%)	861	327	127	47	1362

Table 57 Comparison of mothers' experience this pregnancy with previous one by whether labour was spontaneous or induced

| | Induced this time | | Spontaneous this time | |
| | Last time | | Last time | |
	Induced	Spontaneous	Induced	Spontaneous
	%	%	%	%
Pregnancy this time:				
Easier	27	19	31	24
More difficult	31	38	23	29
About the same	34	34	40	40
Other comment	8	9	6	7
	%	%	%	%
Length of labour this time:				
Shorter	66	68	64	56
Longer	18	18	19	23
Same	16	13	16	21
Other comment	—	1	1	—
	%	%	%	%
Pain this time:				
Better	29	34	39	30
Worse	44	35	31	35
Same	26	30	28	34
Other comment	1	1	2	1
	%	%	%	%
Way looked after this time:				
Better	28	43	32	31
Worse	12	11	11	13
Same	58	45	56	54
Other comment	2	1	1	2
	%	%	%	%
Experience – altogether:				
This time better	41	43	55	43
This time worse	22	23	14	19
Same	35	32	29	36
Other comment	2	2	2	2
	%	%	%	%
This baby:				
More easy	42	44	47	49
More difficult	26	23	22	21
Same	31	31	31	30
Other comment	1	2	—	—
Number of mothers *(= 100%)*	143	159	263	734

time, in relation to mothers' assessments of their experiences, are shown in *Table 57*.

Four pairs of comparisons are possible. Pregnancies were more often reported as easier this time if labour was induced last time. The difference was significant if labour was spontaneous this time, and was in the same direction if it was induced. This is probably because labour is more often induced if the woman has toxaemia of pregnancy and if she is admitted to hospital during pregnancy. The other two comparisons are not significant but are in the direction that supports this hypothesis.

Since induced labours were, on average, shorter than ones that started spontaneously, it was expected that the proportion who thought it was shorter this time would be highest among those induced this time but whose labour started spontaneously last time, and lowest among those whose labour was spontaneous this time and induced last time. In fact the group that stood out was those whose labours started spontaneously both times. They had least variability in that a relatively high proportion thought their labour was a similar length on the two occasions, and the ratio of those who thought it was shorter this time to those who thought it longer was lower for this group than for the other three. When mothers were asked why they thought their labour was longer or shorter this time, induction was preceived as contributing to a shorter labour by almost twice as many women as thought it made it longer, 11 per cent compared with 6 per cent.

For pain, two of the four comparisons had significant differences. Among those who had labours that started spontaneously this time, more of those who were induced last time said it was better this time than of those whose previous labour had been spontaneous. Then, comparing the two groups who had an induced labour last time, they more often felt it was better this time if it had started spontaneously. Both these differences point towards a more painful labour when it was induced. The other two differences are in the opposite direction but are not statistically significant. So on balance the data suggest that induced labour is more painful. And 10 per cent of mothers perceived induction as making their labour more painful compared with 2 per cent who thought it made it less.

Those most likely to feel they had been looked after better this time were those who had induced labours this time and a spontaneous one previously, whereas in their overall assessments it was the opposite group (with a spontaneous labour this time but an induction last time) who compared their recent experience most favourably. There were no significant differences in their comparisons of the babies as being more easy or difficult.

Altogether comparisons suggest that other aspects of their experience rather than an induced or a spontaneous labour were usually of overriding importance, but that in general induced labours were probably perceived as rather more painful.

Choices

Those who had had an induction were asked if they felt they could have refused to have an induction if they had not wanted one, and then if they would say they had a choice about being induced or not. Rather more, 54 per cent, felt they could have refused one than said they had a choice about it, 34 per cent. The proportion who felt they had a choice was higher, 57 per cent, of those who said they were induced because they were overdue than among those who were induced because of high blood pressure or toxaemia, 31 per cent, or because of anxieties about the baby, 29 per cent. This proportion was 42 per cent among those who said they were induced so that the baby could be born at a convenient time.

Rather more middle- than working-class women felt they could have refused an induction, and the proportion who felt they had a choice varied in the same direction but was not statistically significant. The data are in *Table 58*.

It may be that middle-class women have higher expectations, so more of them feel that there should be opportunities for discussion and involvement. Then, even when doctors respond and give some of them a chance to express their views, there are still as many proportionally who feel dissatisfied. If this is so, the relative lack of difference arises because of two conflicting trends which virtually cancel each other out. This explanation is supported by data from other studies. Buchan and Richardson (1973) found a clear social-class gradient in the length of general practitioner consultations, and data from a study of general practitioners consultations with the elderly (Cartwright and O'Brien 1976) showed that more problems were discussed at consultations with middle-class patients, who tended to ask more questions.

All mothers were asked: 'If there is any doubt about which of two things a doctor should do for you, would you prefer him to decide

Table 58 Social class and choices about induction

	Social class						All mothers
	I Profes-sional	II Inter-mediate	III Skilled		IV & V Semi- and Un- skilled	Unclas-sified	
			Non-manual	Manual			
Proportion who felt they could have re-fused induction	66%	63%	57%	51%	46%	59%	54%
Proportion who felt they had a choice about being induced	31%	44%	37%	35%	24%	45%	34%
Number of mothers whose labour was induced (= 100%)	42	79	51	227	114	22	535

without telling you or would you rather he explained and let you choose?' The great majority of mothers, 81 per cent, said they would rather he explained and let them choose. Some of their comments were: 'I'd prefer to choose myself but I'd listen to his judgement'; 'I'd want to know. I'm not frightened when I know what to expect. I wouldn't want to be in ignorance. I don't worry when I'm aware of what's happening'; 'Because he might choose the wrong thing for me. I would want to decide for myself, and if anything did happen to me it would be my fault as I'd made up my own mind about it.'

One in eight would prefer the doctor to decide: 'I wouldn't want to worry and wonder whether I should have chosen the other one.' The rest made other comments: 'I'd ask him to explain and then I'd ask him what he thought I should do. I trust their judgement. As far as I'm concerned they've got all the experience, they know all the ins and outs.'

Although there was a clear trend with social class, with the proportion who said they would prefer the doctor to decide increasing from 7 per cent of those in social class I to 17 per cent in social class V, the most important finding in Table 59 is that three-quarters or more of women in all social classes said they would prefer the doctor to explain and let them choose.

Table 59 Social class and preference about decision making

	Social class							All mothers
	I Profes- sional	II Inter- mediate	III Skilled		IV Semi- skilled	V Un- skilled	Unclas- sified	
			Non- manual	Manual				
	%	%	%	%	%	%	%	%
Prefer doctor to decide	7	11	15	12	16	17	12	12
Let mother choose	84	81	76	83	76	80	81	81
Other comment	9	8	9	5	8	3	7	7
Number of mothers *(= 100%)*	196	369	239	852	310	113	94	2173

In conclusion

There is no doubt that most women think that spontaneous labour is preferable. Generally, women are conservative in that they tend to opt for the things they have experienced. This holds particularly for home births but also for hospital births and for having or not having epidural analgesia. It does not hold for those who had an induction, mainly because induction was perceived as 'unnatural'.

It is clear that many women do not have the choices and information they would like. Four-fifths would prefer to be involved in the decision-making process, but only a third of those who were induced felt they had a choice: 'They never said owt about it. They just said come in'; 'They never asked me – they just do it.' To make appropriate choices people need adequate information, and the majority of mothers wanted more information about some aspects of their care or about the childbearing process. Two-fifths of those who were induced wanted more information about that.

One surprising finding is that the most common source of infor- mation about the process of having a baby for women having their first pregnancy was books. Classes were the next most common source of information, and they were said to be the most helpful source of information by over a quarter of women having their first baby.

It is in relation to their sources of information that social class differences were greatest. Women in social class V depended largely on discussion with relatives and friends. Working-class women felt less well-informed than middle-class ones, and this was reflected in their desire for additional information. Although there was some indication that the minority view that women would prefer *not* to have much information or to be involved in decision making was more prevalent among the lower social classes, the main finding is that working-class women, like middle-class ones, want to be informed, but they are less successful in obtaining information.

7 Views and experiences of obstetricians

In this chapter, induction and other aspects of childbearing are considered from a different viewpoint, that of consultant obstetricians – the most senior doctors concerned with policy in relation to obstetric care. What do they see as the advantages and disadvantages of induction? What is their policy about it and other aspects of obstetric care, and how much do these policies vary between consultants? These are the questions examined here.

Perceived advantages and disadvantages of induction

At the pilot stage of this study, obstetricians were asked open questions about the advantages and disadvantages of induction. Many mentioned circumstances in which it was an advantage or disadvantage, and it was also clear that they saw various advantages and disadvantages for the various groups of people involved – the babies, mothers, obstetricians, midwives, and administrators. In the main study they were therefore asked specific questions about the basic effect on each of these groups – the perinatal mortality rate for babies, the pleasantness of pregnancy and labour for mothers, job satisfaction for obstetricians and midwives, and the ease of running maternity hospitals or departments for administrators. Replies are in *Table 60*.

Four-fifths of the obstetricians thought that the increase in inductions in the last few years had contributed to the fall in the perinatal mortality rate. This would appear to be the main advantage of induction in the obstetricians' eyes. Few, 3 per cent, felt it had slowed

Table 60   Obstetricians' views on the advantages and disadvantages of induction

Effect of increase in inductions	Perinatal mortality rate	Experience of labour and pregnancy for women	Job satis-faction for obstetricians	Job satis-faction for midwives	Running of maternity hospitals and departments
	%	%	%	%	%
Better	79	40	45	35	50
Worse	3	23	2	14	21
No effect	10	34	52	48	28
Other comment	—	3	1	2	1
Don't know	8	—	—	1	—

Number of obstetricians
(= 100%)   379*

* A small proportion, less than 2 per cent, did not answer some of these questions. They have been omitted when calculating percentages.

down the rate of fall in the perinatal mortality rate. Nearly half, 45 per cent, thought it had increased the job satisfaction of obstetricians. Some reasons given for this were: 'Deliveries are now more likely in "office hours" on days of mutual convenience'; 'Intensive monitoring leading to optimum quality child'; 'One is able to give patients more care when labour and delivery is planned'; 'Better results – happier mothers – tidier department'; 'Any procedure which benefits patients and their babies must increase job satisfaction.'

Less than half, two-fifths, thought it had made the experience of labour and pregnancy more pleasant for women, and almost a quarter thought it had made it worse. The main reason for thinking it pleasanter was that it made labour shorter. Other reasons were: 'Domestic arrangements easier'; 'Less fear of prolonged and distressing labour ending in a difficult delivery'; 'Planning and monitoring inducing confidence'; 'Many women like to know when their baby is going to arrive and they feel that an easier birth is achieved by preventing the baby from growing too big.'

Comments from some of those who felt that induction has made the experience of pregnancy and labour less pleasant for women were: 'Although labour shortened by augmentation with oxytocic drip, contractions are probably more intense and painful'; 'Women who have labour induced often feel a sense of failure'; 'No-one can claim that an intravenous drip is pleasant'; 'When inductions are performed freely for non-medical indications, patients feel that they are being interfered with unnecessarily and satisfaction from their reproductive competence is denied them.' Half felt it had made the running of

Table 61   Views of obstetricians on effect of
induction at term for non-medical reasons

	%
Caesarean section	
More likely if induced	37
Less likely if induced	10
No difference	51
Other comment	2
	%
Development of jaundice in baby	
More likely if induced	52
Less likely if induced	—
No difference	45
Other comment	3
	%
Development of significant jaundice in baby	
More likely if induced	25
Less likely if induced	1
No difference	72
Other comment	2
	%
*Forceps**	
More likely if induced	15
Less likely if induced	21
No difference	63
Other comment	1
	%
Length of labour	
Shorter if induced	69
Longer if induced	8
No difference	20
Other comment	3
	%
*Pain in labour**	
More painful if induced	35
Less painful if induced	3
No difference	58
Other comment	4
	%
Hypoxia	
More likely if induced	13
Less likely if induced	23
No difference	60
Other comment	4
*Number of obstetricians (= 100%)***	379

* Assuming an epidural is not given.
** Between 7 per cent and 11 per cent did not
answer the questions and have been omitted.

Table 62 Views of obstetricians on other effects of induction for non-medical reasons

	%
Relationship between mothers and babies	
No effect	65
Uncertain if any effect	28
Some effect	
beneficial	2
harmful	5
	%
Baby's development and growth	
No effect	68
Uncertain if any effect	20
Some effect	
beneficial	1
harmful	7
Other comment	4
	%
The mother's health	
No effect	70
Uncertain if any effect	13
Some effect	
beneficial	2
harmful	12
Other comment	3
*Number of obstetricians (= 100%)**	379

* Between 4 per cent and 7 per cent did not answer the questions and have been omitted.

maternity hospitals or departments easier, but a substantial minority, a fifth, held the opposite view.

Views on one aspect were related to views on others: for instance, 89 per cent of those who thought it had improved the experience of labour and pregnancy for women believed that it had also contributed to the fall in the perinatal mortality rate compared with 80 per cent of those who thought it had not made any difference for women and 60 per cent of those who thought it had made the experience less pleasant for women. So there appeared to be a halo effect; if advantages were seen in one aspect, they were more likely to perceive the effect as favourable in other respects.

120   The Dignity of Labour?

The views of obstetricians on various specific effects of induction at term for non-medical reasons are shown in *Table 61*. The points of greatest agreement were that induction did not affect the development of significant jaundice in the baby (nearly three-quarters said this) and that labour was shorter if induced (two-thirds held this view). Around three-fifths thought that induction made no difference to the use of forceps, to pain in labour, or to the development of hypoxia in the baby. Among those who thought that induction did have an effect on pain in labour, there was a high level of consensus that it made it more painful, but views were more evenly divided on the direction of the effect of Caesarean section, forceps, and hypoxia.

Obstetricians were also asked if they thought that induction for non-medical reasons was likely to affect the relationship between mothers and babies, the baby's development and growth, and the mother's health in any way. Replies are shown in *Table 62*. The majority, two-thirds, did not think it would have any effect; but a sizeable minority, of between one in eight and one in four, were uncertain and, among the few who thought it did have an effect, more felt it would be harmful rather than beneficial.

Policy on induction

Earlier (on page 17) it was shown that consultants' estimates of the proportion of births under their care that were induced varied: 3 per cent of consultants thought they did 10 per cent or less while 5 per cent estimated 50 per cent or more. Forty-two per cent thought it was between 20 per cent and 30 per cent. And the estimated average proportion was 28 per cent. As expected, their views on the advantages were clearly related to the proportion of inductions performed in their units. This is shown in *Table 63*.

There was some indication that consultants whose units induced 30 per cent or more of the births were more likely to use electrical monitoring of the fetal heart routinely than those whose units carried out a lower proportion of inductions (21 per cent of the former used it routinely, 13 per cent of the latter, a difference that might occur by chance). But the availability of ultrasound for cephalometry and facilities for fetal blood sampling in labour appeared to be unrelated to the level of induction. Overall, 17 per cent of the obstetricians said electrical monitoring of the fetal heart was used routinely in their units, 48 per cent that ultrasound for cephalometry was available in the same

Table 63 Level of inductions and obstetricians' views on advantages of induction

Proportion believing the increase in inductions has	Level of inductions				
	Less than 20%	20% < 30%	30% < 40%	40% or more	Inade- quate
Contributed to the fall in the perinatal mortality rate	65%	76%	95%	87%	76%
Made labour and pregnancy more pleasant for women	31%	39%	46%	46%	40%
Increased job satisfaction for obstetricians	40%	44%	48%	58%	32%
Increased job satisfaction for midwives	31%	34%	33%	51%	21%
Made running of maternity hospitals and departments easier	42%	47%	57%	58%	63%
Number of obstetricians (= 100%)	75	147	83	49	25

building for all who needed it, and 70 per cent that there were facilities for fetal blood sampling in labour.

When asked if there would be more or fewer inductions proportionately among the births in their care if they had more resources, the great majority, 90 per cent, said it would not make any difference, 4 per cent said they would do more, and 6 per cent that they would do fewer.

Additional resources that could lead to more inductions were modern monitoring equipment, epidurals, staff, anaesthetists trained to do epidurals, better-trained nurses, and more beds, while those that would lead other obstetricians to do fewer were ultrasound monitoring, better conditions at night, placental function tests, twenty-four hour intensive care coverage, and more experienced midwives and medical staff.

It is difficult to identify a clear-cut policy on induction since decisions about whether and when to induce are likely to depend on many different facets of a particular situation. In an attempt to get

Table 64   Level of inductions by stage at which induction would be suggested

Stage at which induction would be suggested	Level of inductions					All obstetricians
	Less than 20%	20% < 30%	30% < 40%	40% or more	Inadequate	
	%	%	%	%	%	%
Within 7 days of EDD*	1	2	20	15	8	8
7, 8, 9 days after EDD	16	22	32	29	29	24
10, 11, 12 days after EDD	33	40	30	36	38	36
13, 14, 15 days after EDD	28	21	10	10	13	18
16–20 days after EDD	7	} 1	} 2	—	—	2
21 days or more after EDD	—	}	}	—	—	1
Never without other indications	8	9	5	2	4	6
Other answers	7	5	1	8	8	5
Number of obstetricians (= 100%)	75	147	83	48	24	377

* Expected date of delivery.

some indication of the *stage* at which obstetricians would consider induction, a relatively common situation was described and as many of the relevant criteria as seemed appropriate identified. Obstetricians were asked: 'If a woman of twenty-two is having her first baby and is sure of her dates, at what stage would you suggest induction, if there were no other medical or social indications other than prolonged pregnancy and you were certain about the maturity of the fetus?' A third said they would do so within the ten days after the expected date of delivery, just over a third would do so on the tenth, eleventh, or twelfth days, and a quarter would leave it for longer than that or said they would never induce without other indications. Five per cent gave other answers.

As might be expected, those with a relatively high level of induction were more likely to say they would suggest induction at a comparatively early stage. This can be seen from *Table 64.*

The stage at which they would suggest an induction was also related to their views about the advantages of induction. Among those who thought that the increase in induction had contributed to the fall in the perinatal mortality rate, 36 per cent said they would suggest induction within the ten days after the expected date of delivery compared with 15 per cent of other obstetricians.

To try to obtain some picture of non-medical situations in which obstetricians might consider induction, they were asked whether they would agree to, or recommend, induction in the series of circumstances shown in *Table 65*.

Table 65 Some circumstances in which obstetricians would agree to or recommend induction

	Proportion who would agree to or recommend induction in the three days before EDD
A woman having her first baby is certain of her dates, obstetric conditions are favourable, and the woman requests induction three days before EDD. There are no medical indications but the woman requests it so that the baby would be born before her mother goes back to Australia.	46%
A woman having her first baby, is certain of her dates, and obstetric conditions are favourable, and	
(a) there are no medical indications but fairly acute staff shortages at nights and at weekends;	21%
(b) the woman is anxious and you feel that induction may relieve her anxiety but there are no other medical indications;	42%
(c) the woman wants an epidural and the staff responsible for epidurals are not usually on duty at nights or weekends but there are no other indications.	37%
A woman is having her *third* baby, is certain of her dates and obstetric conditions are favourable, and	
(a) the woman has a long and difficult journey to hospital, but there are no other indications;	64%
(b) the woman has a history of precipitate labour but no other indications.	71%
Number of obstetricians (= 100%)	379

Of the six situations described there was most agreement over not recommending induction because of staff shortages. Only a fifth said they would do this. At the other end of the scale, seven-tenths would recommend induction if a woman having a third baby had a history of precipitate labour. Obstetricians were almost evenly divided about agreeing to an induction when a woman requested it for social reasons.

While relatively few obstetricians said they would recommend an induction because of fairly acute staff shortages, a much higher proportion, 43 per cent, said that women under their care sometimes had an induction simply to ensure that expert staff (e.g. a paediatrician) would be available when the baby was born.[1] Replies to this question and to the six circumstances in *Table 65* were put together into an 'induction index' which ranged from nil to seven. Those scoring nil would not recommend or advise it in any circumstances; those scoring seven did so in all the circumstances.

The average induction index was 3.2. It fell from 3.4 for those who thought induction had contributed to the fall in the perinatal mortality rate to 2.3 for other obstetricians; it was 3.8 for those who thought it had made the experience of labour and pregnancy more pleasant for mothers and 2.9 for others. It was strongly related to the stage at which they would induce a woman of twenty-two having her first baby, ranging from 5.4 for those who would induce within seven days of the EDD down to 2.2 for those who would wait for thirteen days or more. It rose from 2.9 for those inducing less than 30 per cent to 3.5 for those doing between 30 per cent and 40 per cent, and to 4.3 for those doing 40 per cent or more. Appropriately, it was highly correlated within obstetricians' estimates of the proportion of the induced births under their care that, in the last twelve months, were done for reasons not strictly medical in the sense that neither the woman nor the fetus had a medical indication. This can be seen from *Table 66*, which also shows the distribution of their estimates. The average was 7 per cent.

Rather surprisingly, estimates of the proportion of non-medical inductions were not related to their prediction about whether they would do more or fewer inductions if they had more resources.

Obstetricians were asked whether or not women were always given

---

[1] 'Does a woman under your care ever have an induction simply to ensure that expert staff (e.g. a paediatrician) will be available when the baby is born?'

Table 66 Proportion of induced births in the last twelve months estimated as being done for reasons that were not strictly medical

Proportion of non-medical inductions	%	Average induction index
None	31	1.5
Less than 2%	19	3.0
2% but less than 5%	14	3.6
5% but less than 10%	18	3.9
10% but less than 25%	13	
25% but less than 50%	2	
50% but less than 75%	2	5.0
75% or more	1	
Number of obstetricians *(= 100%)*	361*	

* Three per cent of obstetricians did not answer this question and a further 1 per cent said they did some but did not indicate what proportion. These have been excluded from the table. The average induction index for those who were excluded was 3.4.

a choice about inductions for reasons that were not strictly medical.[2] Seventeen per cent said it never happened that women were induced for reasons that were strictly non-medical, 68 per cent that they were always given a choice, 8 per cent that they were not always given a choice, and 7 per cent gave other answers.

They were also asked who usually explained to the women under their care who were to be induced what was involved in an induction. Many gave more than one answer, but 16 per cent said the consultant only, 3 per cent the registrar only, and 45 per cent the consultant or registrar. Two-thirds mentioned doctors of varying rank only, three out of ten a sister or staff midwife as well as a doctor.

The various methods ever used for induction are shown in *Table 67*. The main method was the combination of A R M and oxytocin. For 83 per cent of the consultants this was the method most often used for inductions under their care.

In general, different aspects of obstetricians' induction policy were related to one another and to their views on the advantages and

[2] 'If there is a possibility of a woman under your care being induced for a reason that is not strictly medical, would you say she is given a choice about this or not?'

Table 67   Methods of induction ever used

	%
ARM only	59
ARM and oxytocin or synthetic oxytocin	98
ARM and prostaglandins	37
Prostaglandins only	28
Oxytocin only	36
Membrane sweep	16
Other	6
Number of obstetricians (= 100%)	362

disadvantages of induction. There is less evidence that induction policy is clearly related to the availability of resources and some apparently conflicting data about this: two-fifths of the obstetricians said that women under their care sometimes had inductions simply to ensure that expert staff would be available at delivery, but less than one in eighteen said they would do fewer inductions if they had more resources.

Acceleration

Apart from induction, women who go into labour spontaneously may have their labour accelerated or augmented, and this too may be done surgically or with drugs or by a combination of the two. Obstetricians were asked to estimate the proportion of births for which they were responsible that were accelerated or augmented but not induced, and the proportion who were given drugs (oxytocin, synthetic oxytocin, or prostaglandins) either to accelerate or induce labour. Replies are shown in *Table 68*, alongside their estimates of the proportion induced.

The proportion of labours that were accelerated but not induced would seem to be appreciably less than the proportion that were induced, the averages being 28 per cent for inductions, and 17 per cent for accelerations. The average proportion given drugs for either induction or acceleration was 36 per cent, so acceleration probably accounts for over a quarter of the use of oxytocin or prostaglandins. Two-thirds of the consultants who answered this question estimated that at least 30 per cent of the women were given these drugs either to induce or to accelerate their labour. Just over one-third put their induction rate as high as that.

Table 68   Estimates of the proportion induced, accelerated, and of those given drugs to induce or accelerate

	Proportion induced	Proportion accelerated but not induced	Proportion given drugs to induce or accelerate
	%	%	%
Less than 5%	1	13	2
5% < 10%	2	23	4
10% < 20%	18	35	10
20% < 30%	42	17	18
30% < 40%	23	6	26
40% < 50%	9	5	22
50% < 60%	4	} 1	10
60% < 70%	} 1		6
70% or more			2
Number of obstetricians making estimate (= 100%) *354		337	315

* The proportions giving inadequate or inconsistent replies were 7 per cent to the first question, 11 per cent to the second, and 17 per cent to the third.

It might be thought that obstetricians who did a relatively high proportion of inductions might do comparatively fewer accelerations without inductions than their colleagues, since a smaller proportion of their patients would be 'at risk' to this possibility. An alternative hypothesis might be that consultants doing a high proportion of inductions were in favour of intervention and would therefore also do relatively more accelerations without induction. In practice the induction rate did not seem to be associated either positively or negatively with the proportion they accelerated but did not induce. But, as expected, the proportion estimating that 50 per cent or more of the women under their care were given oxytocin or prostaglandins rose with their induction rate from 1 per cent of those inducing less than 20 per cent to 60 per cent with an induction rate of 40 per cent or more.

Epidurals

Another procedure sometimes associated with induction is epidural anaesthesia. Among the 84 per cent of consultants who said that epidurals were given to some of the women under their care, half

Table 69 Association between induction and epidural rates

Proportion of women given epidurals	Level of inductions					All obstetricians
	Less than 20%	20% < 30%	30% < 40%	40% or more	Inadequate	
	%	%	%	%	%	%
None	24 ⎫42	15 ⎫36	14 ⎫25	10 ⎫16	20	16
Less than 5%	18 ⎭	21 ⎭	11 ⎭	6 ⎭	10	16
5% < 10%	8	11	16	10	10	11
10% < 25%	26	26	31	41	10	28
25% < 50%	14	17	16	19	15	16
50% < 75%	7	6	10	8	5	7
75% or more	—	1	—	4	10	2
Some: inadequate how many	3	3	2	2	20	4
Number of obstetricians (= 100%)	72	144	81	49	20	366

Table 70 Obstetricians' views of the advantages and disadvantages of epidurals

Effect of use of epidurals	Experience of labour and pregnancy for women	Job satisfaction for obstetricians	Job satisfaction for midwives
	%	%	%
Better	89	63	55
Worse	2	4	13
No effect	6	31	27
Other comment	2	1	3
Don't know	1	1	2
Number of obstetricians (= 100%)	355	349	349

thought that women were more likely to be given an epidural if they were induced. (The others thought it did not make any difference, apart from 1 per cent who thought the induced were less likely to have one.) And a third thought that if a woman wanted an epidural then she was more likely to be induced (none thought induction was less likely in this circumstance). *Table 69* shows the association between their estimated induction and epidural rates for the obstetricians. It is positive, but not very strong ($r = +0.13$, $p < .05$).

In terms of their effect on the mothers, obstetricians were more in favour of epidurals than inductions in that a higher proportion of them felt they had a good effect. This can be seen by comparing *Table 70* with *Table 60*. In addition, of those already doing some epidurals, two-thirds said they would do more if they had more resources. (All the others, apart from one, said it would not make any difference.)

Most, three-quarters of those involved with epidurals said that nulliparas, women having their first pregnancy, were more likely to have them, 3 per cent that they were less likely to do so, the others that it

Table 71   Level of epidurals and midwives' involvement in 'topping up' and the choice offered to women

	Proportion given epidurals					All obste-tricians
	Less than 5%	5% < 10%	10% < 25%	25% < 50%	50% or more	
	%	%	%	%	%	%
Proportion of 'topping up' done by midwives						
None	50	31	18	13	10	24
Less than 50%	9	18	16	16	13	14
50% < 75%	15	20	17	21	32	20
75% < 90%	9	8	20	14	3	13
90% or more	17	23	29	36	42	29
	%	%	%	%	%	%
Choice of women in relation to epidurals						
Offered to all women	—	7	17	37	84	24
Given to those who ask for it	29	21	28	20	13	24
Given for medical reasons only	32	29	7	3	—	13
Given to those who ask and for medical reasons	10	22	28	18	—	18
Other	29	21	20	22	3	21
Number of obstetricians* (= 100%)	57	42	103	60	32	319

* Eleven per cent did not answer the question on 'topping up', and 3 per cent the one concerning women's choices. They were excluded when the percentages were calculated.

made no difference. For the most part, 85 per cent, anaesthetists were said to be responsible for giving epidurals; 4 per cent said obstetricians were responsible, and 11 per cent that it was both. The epidural rate was similar when anaesthetists were solely responsible and when obstetricians were involved. But one thing that increased with the epidural rate was the involvement of midwives in the topping up. Overall, 24 per cent of obstetricians involved with epidurals said that midwives never did the topping up, while, at the other end of the scale, 29 per cent of obstetricians said that midwives did 90 per cent or more of the topping up.[3] The proportion saying midwives never did it fell from 50 per cent of obstetricians when less than 5 per cent of their patients had epidurals, to 10 per cent of those whose epidural rate was 50 per cent or more. And the higher the proportion of epidurals they did, the more likely they were to offer all their patients a choice about this.[4] (See *Table 71*.)

Episiotomies

The other aspect of obstetric care that obstetricians were asked about was episiotomies. They were asked to estimate the proportion of

Table 72 Proportion of episiotomies

	%
Less than 10%	—
10% < 20%	2
20% < 30%	9
30% < 40%	10
40% < 50%	8
50% < 60%	18
60% < 70%	15
70% < 80%	20
80% < 90%	10
90% or more	8
Number of obstetricians (= 100%)	332

[3] 'When epidurals need to be topped up, in what percentage of instances would you say it is done by midwives?'
[4] 'What choice do women in your care have about epidurals – is it offered to all women, given to those who ask for it, given for medical reasons only (other – specify)?'

deliveries under their care at which episiotomies were performed. The distribution is shown in *Table 72*. It was not correlated with their induction rate but was positively related to the proportion of epidurals given in the departments (r = + 0.26, p < .001).

These findings suggest that epidurals lead to a need for episiotomies rather than episiotomies and induction arising from a general interventionist policy on the part of obstetricians.

Some differences between obstetricians

Is it possible to identify any characteristics of obstetricians that are associated with their induction policy – other than their perceptions of the advantages and disadvantages of induction? Thirteen per cent of the obstetricians were women, and there was some suggestion that the women's induction rate was slightly lower than the men's (27 per cent of the women compared with 39 per cent of the men said that 30 per cent or more of the women under their care were induced). Women doctors were no more or less likely than men to say that induction had made the experience of labour more pleasant for women, and the induction index of the two sexes was similar.

There was no clear trend of the induction rate with age. If anything,

Table 73   Obstetricians' date of birth and induction rate

	Obstetricians' date of birth					
	1915 or earlier	1916–20	1921–5	1926–30	1931–5	1936 or later
	%	%	%	%	%	%
Induction rate						
Less than 10%	4	7	4	3	3	—
10% < 20%	17	22	21	22	10	18
20% < 30%	54	39	31	38	40	48
30% < 40%	13	20	20	22	35	26
40% < 50%	6 } 12	5 } 12	18 } 24	12 } 15	8 } 12	5 } 8
50% or more	6	7	6	3	4	3
Average induction index	3.2	3.7	4.0	2.9	2.9	2.7
Number of obstetricians* (= 100%)	53	60	52	72	77	64

* Seven per cent who did not answer the question have been excluded when calculating percentages.

Table 74 Views of obstetricians, with university and NHS appointments, on induction

| | Appointment | |
	University	NHS
	%	%
Caesarean section		
More likely if induced	49	35
Less likely if induced	2*	11
No difference	49	52
Other comment	—	2
	%	%
Forceps (assuming no epidural)		
More likely if induced	19	14
Less likely if induced	7*	23
No difference	74	62
Other comment	—	1
	%	%
Hypoxia		
More likely if induced	23	12
Less likely if induced	12*	24
No difference	53	61
Other comment	12	3
	%	%
Effect of induction on relationship between mother and baby		
None	55	66
Uncertain	34	27
Some		
beneficial	—	2
harmful	9	4
Other comment	2	1
	%	%
Effect of induction on baby's development		
None	55	70
Uncertain	27	18
Some		
beneficial	—	2
harmful	11	6
Other comment	7	4
		(continued)

| | Appointment | |
	University	NHS
	%	%
Labour		
More painful if induced	45	34
Less painful if induced	3	4
No difference	52	58
Other comment	—	4
	%	%
Effect of induction on mother's health		
None	43*	74
Uncertain	34*	10
Some		
beneficial	—	2
harmful	16	12
Other comment	7	2
*Number of obstetricians*** (= 100%)	46	333

* Difference significant (p < .05).
** Those who gave inadequate responses have been omitted when calculating the percentages.

those born between 1921 and 1925 (in their early fifties at the time of the survey) appeared to have a relatively high induction rate and a high induction index (see *Table 73*). Possibly older obstetricians are more conservative and less inclined to adopt new techniques. Younger doctors may be the first to adopt them and the first to give them up. Certainly more of those born since 1925 said they were doing proportionally fewer inductions currently than they were two years previously: 11 per cent compared with 4 per cent of the older doctors.

Doctors with university rather than NHS appointments estimated that they induced a slighly smaller proportion of their patients. The proportion who said they induced 40 per cent or more was 4 per cent of those with a university appointment compared with 15 per cent of the others. This is in line with the finding from the mothers that those in 'teaching' hospitals were less likely to be induced than those in 'non-teaching' ones.

Obstetricians with university appointments also tended to be less enthusiastic about induction than those with NHS appointments. The former were less likely to feel that there were advantages, and more likely to be uncertain about possible after-effects. Some differences are shown in *Table 74*. They are all in the same direction, but only those marked with an asterisk reached a level of statistical significance.

However, it was not that obstetricians with university appointments were anti-interventionist or against high technology obstetrics in other respects. They give epidurals to a higher proportion of their patients than did other obstetricians. This is shown in *Table 75*.

Table 75   Proportion of patients receiving epidurals for obstetricians with university and NHS appointments

	Appointment	
	University	NHS
	%	%
None	—	19
Less than 5%	4	18
5% < 10%	4	13
10% < 25%	31	29
25% < 50%	46	13
50% or more	15	8
Number of obste-		
tricians (= 100%)	46	306

One obvious reason for this is that those with university appointments have more facilities. A much smaller proportion of them said more epidurals would be given in their unit if more resources were available: 43 per cent compared with 73 per cent of other obstetricians. And fewer of those in university posts said obstetricians had responsibility for giving epidurals: 4 per cent against 16 per cent.

Earlier it was shown that the higher the proportion of epidurals given, the greater the likelihood of midwives doing the 'topping-up'. This would lead to the expectation that midwives would do more of the 'topping-up' in units headed by an obstetrician in a university post. In practice there was no difference between the two groups on this – further evidence of greater facilities in terms of more medical staff being available in the teaching units.

Obstetricians with university appointments were also more likely to have access to other facilities such as ultra-sound, amniocentesis, and

Table 76   Facilities available for obstetricians in university and NHS appointments

	Appointment		All obste-tricians
	University	NHS	
Ultra-sound for cephalometry available in same building if needed	80%	44%	48%
Amniocentesis available for all necessary pregnancies	98%	91%	92%
Facilities for fetal blood sampling in labour available	89%	68%	70%
Electrical monitoring of the fetal heart used routinely	27%	15%	17%
Number of obstetricians (= 100%)	46	333	379

fetal blood-sampling facilities. The figures are in *Table 76*.

Altogether the differences in availability of resources between obstetricians in NHS and university posts are considerably greater than the identified differences in attitudes.

There is the additional complication that those in university posts are, as a group, younger than those in NHS posts. Only a fifth of the former were born in 1925 or earlier compared with almost half, 47 per cent, of the others. When age is held constant, the differences with type of appointment in their practices and views on induction still persist, although not all are statistically significant.

In conclusion

The data from the consultant obstetricians suggest that the level of induction is not likely to rise greatly in the future and is more likely to decline. This conclusion is based on the fact that younger obstetricians were more likely than older ones to say they were currently doing fewer inductions than they were two years previously, and on the fact that younger doctors and those in university appointments, the groups most likely to be the trend-setters, were doing slightly smaller proportions of inductions than others. But both these effects were small and, by themselves, would only indicate a very small change. Another small indication that inductions are slightly more likely to decrease rather than increase is that, if anything, slighly more obstetricians said

Table 77   Obstetricians' estimates of the proportion of women who would prefer various arrangements

Estimated proportion of women who would prefer procedure	Inductions	Epidurals	Home births
	%	%	%
80% +	5	3	—
70% < 80%	6	4	—
60% < 70%	5	9	1
50% < 60%	14	13	2
40% < 50%	10	12	—
30% < 40%	12	13	2
20% < 30%	17	20	5
10% < 20%	12	15	15
5% < 10%	11	5	26
Less than 5%	8	6	49
Average proportion	36%	36%	9%
Number of obstetricians (= 100%)	318	314	322

they would do fewer inductions if they had more resources than said they would do more: 6 per cent against 4 per cent, an insignificant difference but one in striking contrast to their replies about the effect of more resources on their epidural rate. Two-thirds of the obstetricians already doing some epidurals said they would do more if more resources were available.

In terms of anxieties about 'high technology' obstetrics, the likely increase in the epidural rate might be seen as posing more of a threat to 'natural' childbirth than induction. In this context it is relevant to consider obstetricians' views of women's attitudes and preferences. It will be recalled that 89 per cent of obstetricians thought the increase in epidurals had made the experience of childbearing more pleasant for women compared with 40 per cent who thought this about the increase in inductions, while the proportion who thought the procedures had made the experience less pleasant were 2 per cent for epidurals and 23 per cent for inductions. Obstetricians were asked what proportions of women would prefer to have an induction, an epidural, or home birth if they were given a choice.[5] Replies are given in *Table 77*.

[5] 'What proportion of all women do you think would opt to have their labour induced if they were given a choice shortly before their EDD?' 'What proportion would choose to have an epidural?' 'What proportion would prefer to have their babies at home?'

Rather surprisingly, in view of their other comments, their estimates of the proportion of women who would prefer an induction were very similar to their estimates of the proportion who would prefer an epidural. In both instances the average was 36 per cent. This is in striking contrast to their estimates of the proportion who would prefer a home birth. The average for this was 9 per cent.

Comparing these estimates with the proportions of mothers who said they would prefer these arrangements if they were to have another baby, obstetricians would appear to greatly overestimate the popularity of induction, since only 8 per cent of mothers said they would prefer this. And even for those who had an induction for their last labour, this proportion was only 17 per cent. They also overestimated, but not to such a great extent, the proportion who said they would like an epidural. This was 16 per cent of all mothers, but was substantially higher, 63 per cent, of those who had had an epidural. In contrast, they underestimated the proportion who would opt for a home birth. This was 18 per cent of all mothers and 91 per cent of those who had had a home birth.

Clearly many, but not all, obstetricians are unaware of the extent of the antipathy towards induction among childbearing women, and do not realize the extent of the 'demand' for home births.

8 Views and experiences of midwives

Most babies born in this country are delivered by midwives. The proportion on this survey was three-quarters. It was two-thirds of the induced labours, just over three-quarters of those that started spontaneously. So, while midwives do not have responsibility for initiating induction, they have wide experience of both induced and non-induced labour and the aftermath. What are their views of the advantages and disadvantages of induction? How do their views and experiences compare with those of obstetricians? To try to answer these questions, 388 midwives working in hospitals where the mothers in the study had their live babies were interviewed.

The advantages and disadvantages of induction

Like the obstetricians, the main advantage of induction perceived by the midwives was that it had contributed to the fall in the perinatal mortality rate. But fewer midwives than obstetricians held this view, 66 per cent compared with 79 per cent, and more midwives thought it had not had any effect on this, 24 per cent against 10 per cent. The figures for the midwives are in *Table 78*, which shows that almost half of them, 47 per cent, thought that the increase in induction had made the experience of labour and pregnancy worse for women. It may be recalled that just under a quarter of the obstetricians held this view.

Some comments from the midwives about the ways in which they felt it had made experiences less pleasant for mothers were:

Table 78 Midwives' views on the advantages and disadvantages of induction

Effect of increase in inductions	Perinatal mortality rate	Experience of labour and pregnancy for women	Job satis-faction for obstetricians	Job satis-faction for midwives	Running of maternity hospitals and departments
	%	%	%	%	%
Better	66	21	49	18	34
Worse	3	47	2	32	32
No effect	24	22	36	45	28
Other comment	—	9	3	3	4
Don't know	7	1	10	2	2
Number of midwives (= 100%)			388		

'I feel the mothers feel they've been cheated in a sense. The amount of sedation that has to be given means that half of them when they come round are not actually aware of the baby's birth.'

'A terrible psychological effect – the relaxation they learn is no good to them when they are induced – they don't go into labour naturally.'

'They're not in labour so long – but the contractions are much more severe – a gradual labour is more pleasant.'

'It's not a normal experience. I wouldn't like to be induced. Everything is a bit rushed for them in labour. It's quite frightening for them – even just setting the drip up.'

'No woman can find it pleasant to have her membranes artificially ruptured and must prefer to have a natural childbirth – more sense of achievement.'

'Mainly from a psychological point of view. Women don't like machinery and would rather have a normal labour.'

'I think they feel something very clinical is happening to them, like an operation. It's not something natural any more.'

'I've worked in the community for a long time. I had mothers coming home from hospital. I found they were quite frightened of the machinery. If it was for the safety of the baby they would put up with it, but I don't think they found it pleasant.'

Some contrary views from those who thought it had made the experience more pleasant were:

'It's stopped the total exhaustion of women in labour. They're not in labour so long. Strong contractions straightaway, but better analgesia.'

'A shorter labour – can arrange family and husband matters better now.'

'Better because it's shorter, therefore mother not getting so tired. But some hospitals don't prepare the mothers enough for what's going to happen.'

'If you go about it in the right way. We were taught anything can be overcome by the personal touch.'

More midwives thought it had detracted from the job satisfaction for their profession than thought it had added to it. Some reasons for the more common view were:

'We have to rely more on doctors. We're not practitioners in our own right. Before, women would go into labour just with the midwife's help. Now, far more reliance on technology and expertise of obstetricians.'

'No job satisfaction at all. It's like a production line. I don't like working in the labour ward – everything is so quick and so rushed.'

'It's more a mechanical process now – less depends on the midwife's judgement. It's taken out of our hands a bit now.'

'You don't look after your patients in the same way. I used to like getting mothers up to walk around. Now we don't do this – it's all machinery and bed pans.'

'We tend to become mechanical – we forget they are human beings and have feelings and do belong to society. When I do a normal delivery there's more of a link between you and the mothers, and when you deliver an induction mother there isn't the same link.'

But the opposite views were also expressed:

'You see a patient delivered in a day before you go off duty.'

'Well, the patients' labour has been speeded up and the women seem happy and are not left in pain so long.'

'When you're looking after patients who've had an induction you look after her all the way through her labour and direct your whole attention to her. You get to know her better, whereas before we often didn't see a case through.'

'Probably because you're not so worried about the patient dragging on. It's a much more organized programme. You're more aware of what's happening – partly due to the machines now being used.'

'A nurse is always with the patient [with induction] – more contact between nurses and patient. In normal labour the nurse is just popping in and out.'

The midwives were more evenly divided in their views on the effect on the running of a maternity hospital or department. Even so, proportionally more of them than of the obstetricians felt the increase in inductions made the organization more difficult (32 per cent against 21 per cent). Some ways in which it was thought to make organization easier were: 'Because they can plan to have the deliveries more spaced out – not a glut all at once'; 'The patients are usually delivered during the day when there are sufficient staff to cope.' Things that made it more difficult were: 'One has to give more care to the patient, observe more carefully, put them on monitors and drips and supervise these'; 'Because so many are started at about 9 o'clock and they're all going to deliver at around the same time, about 5 o'clock say. Then it's all happening at once'; 'If you're short of staff then it's difficult as you've got so many things to deal with – the rate of drip to regulate, etc. Inductions need a lot more supervising and we're short of staff and space as it is.'

The one effect of the increase in inductions that midwives were not less pessimistic about than obstetricians was its effect on the job satisfaction of obstetricians! Half of them thought it had increased this, whereas the most common view of the obstetricians (held by 52 per cent) was that it had had no effect. Some of the midwives' comments about this were: 'It gives them more work, but they have more to do with the actual patient in labour. It makes them more important'; 'They are so interested in their machines and love their machines. It's helped them to avoid things which they couldn't avoid years ago, but I feel they put machinery first rather than people'; 'They can organize their day better and perhaps not up so much at night.' Other, rather more sympathetic, comments were: 'It has increased their work load and given them more to think about, and the more you have to think about things you get more satisfaction'; 'They're happier because ultimately they're getting much better results.'

As with the obstetricians, their views on the effect of the increase in inductions on one factor tended to be related to their views on other effects. The proportion who thought it had decreased job satisfaction among midwives was 44 per cent of those who thought it had had an adverse effect on the experience of pregnancy and labour for women, compared with 19 per cent of those who thought it had made the experience for women more pleasant (it was 25 per cent of those who thought it had had no effect). But the association is not 'one to one'. So job satisfaction in relation to a particular technique is related to other things besides the reactions of mothers to that technique.

Midwives' views on the effect of induction at term for non-medical reasons are compared with those of obstetricians in *Table 79*. The proportion believing that labour was more painful was almost twice as high among midwives (two-thirds) than among obstetricians (one-third). A higher proportion of midwives than of obstetricians thought that forceps were more likely to be used for induced births – but it was only a minority who held this view. The other main difference between them related to hypoxia: a third of the midwives compared with one in eight of the obstetricians thought that babies were more likely to develop this if labour was induced. When there was a significant difference between them, midwives were more likely to see induction as being disadvantageous except over the development of jaundice in the baby, which more obstetricians thought likely.[1]

Midwives were also rather more likely to think that induction for non-medical reasons might have a deleterious effect on the mother-baby relationship, 10 per cent compared with 5 per cent of obstetricians, and that it might affect the baby's development and health in a harmful way, 11 per cent against 7 per cent. Similar proportions of both groups, around one in eight, thought it likely to have a harmful effect on the mother's health. Descriptions of the way it might be harmful to the relationship between mother and baby were: 'A lot of the mothers and babies have to be separated for the baby to go to a special care unit and I think that's bound to matter'; 'Because the mother had a more painful labour and she has more problems in accepting the baby.' These two mechanisms, separation and more pain, were mentioned by several midwives. Other points were: 'I think it's because we've taken over from nature. I think the process of labour

---

[1] Obstetricians were asked about the development of jaundice and then about the development of 'significant jaundice'. Midwives were only asked the first question, and this is what has been compared. The proportion of obstetricians who thought 'significant jaundice' was more likely after induction was 25 per cent.

Table 79 Views of obstetricians and midwives on effect of induction at term for non-medical reasons

	Obstetricians	Midwives
	%	%
Caesarean section		
More likely if induced	37	33
Less likely if induced	10	12
No difference	51	52
Other comment	2	3
	%	%
Development of jaundice in baby		
More likely if induced	52	42
Less likely if induced	—	1
No difference	45	48
Other comment	3	9
	%	%
*Forceps**		
More likely if induced	15	28
Less likely if induced	21	8
No difference	63	63
Other comment	1	1
	%	%
Length of labour		
Shorter if induced	69	73
Longer if induced	8	11
No difference	20	10
Other comment	3	6
	%	%
*Pain in labour**		
More painful if induced	35	67
Less painful if induced	3	4
No difference	58	23
Other comment	4	6
	%	%
Hypoxia		
More likely if induced	13	35
Less likely if induced	23	7
No difference	60	53
Other comment	4	5
*Number of professionals (= 100%)***	379	388

  * Assuming an epidural is not given.
** Between 7 per cent and 9 per cent did not answer the question and have been omitted.

brings about a feeling, an instinct, that doesn't develop to the full if it's interfered with'; 'They have a bigger relationship problem because they haven't done it themselves. Not so satisfied as if they had given birth the natural way, they feel cheated'; 'The attitudes of mothers – if they want induction then they want to get it over with and the baby is a nuisance.'

This last point, that it was a woman's attitude in wanting an induction that was likely to be associated with a poor relationship, was made by more than one midwife: 'They want to get it over with and it's a nuisance and can bring a lot of depression later on. I always feel that people who want an induction for non-medical reasons don't want their babies.'

The main ways in which non-medical induction might have a harmful effect on the baby's health were that the delivery was likely to be more traumatic and that the baby might be premature, 'if a mistake has been made on the maturity of the baby'. Other possibilities mentioned were jaundice and: 'There's more likely to be brain damage later in life, having too much oxygen. We've yet to see the results in their later life.'

> 'They seem a lot more mucousy and they tend to vomit in the first twenty-four to forty-eight hours. They don't seem to enjoy their food much. I think the greatest risk [of induction] for non-medical reasons is that they are premature babies – I'm not talking about dates. They *act* prematurely, they behave like premature babies often do – often.'

Possible physical effects on the mother were seen as haemorrhages, embolism, painful scar affecting her sex life, or prolapse later on in life (from quick dilation of the cervix). But the most commonly mentioned effect was a psychological one: 'Psychologically she could be affected because the labour has been so rapid the mother hasn't had time to acclimatize to the birth – and they go hysterical. There's nothing you can do; it passes in a few days'; 'Psychologically. Her mental state – she might batter the baby if it's not a natural event.'

> 'Mentally, psychologically, I think that when a woman goes into spontaneous labour she's prepared psychologically and therefore relaxed physically. Regardless of how well induction has been explained to her, I'm sure there's a hormonal effect that makes a woman ready for labour that you can't simulate with induction.'

Some of these comments by midwives about the possible ill-effects of induction, particularly those relating to the long-term effects, merit consideration and possibly investigation. The perception that induction may be associated with depression is supported by findings from this study. But the majority of midwives did not think that induction had these harmful effects. Even so, on balance, midwives had a less rosy view of induction than obstetricians. What of their professional experiences of induction?

Experiences of induction

Midwives were asked to estimate the proportion of births that they were involved in that were induced. When the 17 per cent who said they were not involved with deliveries at all are excluded, the estimated average proportion of inductions is 39 per cent, appreciably and significantly higher than that estimated by the obstetricians. In addition, half the midwives, 49 per cent, said that more inductions were being done among the births in which they were involved than two years ago, 12 per cent said fewer, and 36 per cent the same proportion (the rest made other comments). This contrasts with data from the obstetricians, 20 per cent of whom said they were now doing more, 7 per cent fewer, and 73 per cent the same proportion. And data from HIPE suggest the proportion may, in fact, be falling!

Is it possible that midwives were not always distinguishing between induction and acceleration when making their estimates? Twenty-eight per cent of midwives involved with deliveries estimated that less than 5 per cent of the mothers whose care they were involved in were accelerated but not induced. Only 13 per cent of obstetricians put the proportion as low as that. But the average proportion of estimated accelerations without induction was the same for the two groups: 17 per cent. So too were the proportions they estimated as being given drugs for either induction or acceleration: the average estimate by the midwives was 39 per cent, compared with 36 per cent by obstetricians.

A more plausible explanation for the discrepancy is that midwives included more inductions done by ARM alone in their estimates of the proportion of inductions. Seventeen per cent of midwives compared with only 4 per cent of obstetricians said this was the main method of induction used for the births they were involved with. It may be recalled that mothers reported ARM's for induction or acceleration more often than they were recorded in the medical notes (see page 15). So the data from the three sources indicate that obstetricians may underestimate surgical inductions, and these may also be unrecorded in the medical notes. There is still the puzzle about whether inductions are increasing or declining. This cannot be resolved by a study at a single point in time.

Obstetricians in units with a high proportion of inductions were more likely to see advantages in the procedure than those in units with a low proportion. The association is likely to arise because obstetricians who perceive advantages in a procedure are more likely to adopt it. But midwives are not policy makers in relation to induction. Is there any association for them between the level of induction and their views of the advantages or disadvantages? And, if so, in which direction? In practice, there were no clear trends. Almost two-thirds of the midwives, 63 per cent, said that none of the inductions they had been involved with in the previous twelve months had been done for reasons that were not strictly medical. Less than a third, 30 per cent, of the obstetricians said this. And midwives were less likely than obstetricians to think that women would be induced in the various circumstances listed in *Table 80*.

In addition, 19 per cent of midwives compared with 43 per cent of obstetricians said that inductions were sometimes done simply to ensure that expert staff were available. However, midwives' views on the stage at which a woman having her first baby was likely to be induced[2] were fairly similar to the obstetricians' predictions.

It may be recalled that only 3 per cent of women who were induced did not perceive some medical reason for the induction, whereas on average the obstetricians estimated 7 per cent. It seems unlikely that obstetricians would overestimate the proportion of inductions they were doing simply for non-medical reasons, so the lower estimates from mothers, and the high proportion of midwives who said no inductions were done for non-medical reasons, probably arise either because obstetricians emphasize medical aspects of the situation or because mothers and midwives search for medical reasons and sometimes perceive them when they do not exist.

Midwives were more likely than obstetricians to think that lack of resources limited the number of inductions that were carried out.

[2] 'If a woman of twenty-two is having her first baby and is sure of her dates, at what stage do you think she is most likely to be induced if there are no medical indications other than prolonged pregnancy and the obstetrician is certain about the maturity of the fetus?'

Table 80   Action of obstetricians and views of midwives on probable outcome in various circumstances

	Proportion of obstetricians who would agree to or recommend induction	Proportion of midwives who thought women would be induced
A woman having her first baby is certain of her dates and obstetric conditions are favourable. There are no medical indications but she requests an induction three days before EDD so that the baby will be born before her mother goes back to Australia.	46%	23%
A woman having her first baby is certain of her dates and obstetric conditions are favourable. There are no medical indications but fairly acute staff shortages at nights and weekends.	21%	12%
A woman having her *third* baby is certain of her dates and obstetric conditions are favourable, and she has a long and difficult journey to hospital, but there are no other indications.	64%	15%
Number of professionals (= 100%)	379	310*

* Excluding those not involved with inductions.

Eighteen per cent of them said that they thought more of the births they were involved in would be induced if there were more resources; 3 per cent thought it would lead to fewer inductions. Corresponding proportions for obstetricians were 4 per cent and 6 per cent.

Views and experiences of epidurals

One possible reason for midwives being less enthusiastic than obstetricians about induction is that more midwives dislike high technology medicine. If this is so one would expect them also to be less in favour of epidurals. And this proved to be the case among the minority of midwives, 42 per cent, with experience of epidurals. Fewer midwives than obstetricians thought the use of epidurals had made the experience of labour more pleasant for mothers, 72 per cent compared with 89 per cent; that it had increased job satisfaction for midwives, 26 per cent against 55 per cent; and that it had increased job satisfaction for obstetricians, 39 per cent against 63 per cent. But, whereas with inductions more midwives thought it had improved job satisfaction for obstetricians than thought it had made the experience more pleasant for women (49 per cent compared with 21 per cent), their views on who gained from epidurals were quite different. Over-simplifying, midwives see the high technology of induction as decreasing perinatal mortality and increasing the job satisfaction of obstetricians, while the high technology of epidurals is seen as most beneficial to women in labour. Both were viewed as decreasing the job satisfaction of midwives.

Episiotomies

On average midwives estimated that episiotomies were performed at 60 per cent of the deliveries they were involved with. This is similar to the average proportion estimated by the consultants, but only 49 per cent of the mothers who answered the question said they had been cut. Comments from midwives who said 80 per cent or more of the mothers they were involved with had episiotomies were: 'I think it's a good thing. Women who used not to have them were found to have prolapses later on in life'; 'Sometimes I think they're scissor-happy. Some stretch easily and it's a shame to spoil them. A doctor thought one necessary but I didn't and so he didn't on my advice and it was O. K.'; 'I'm not too keen, it's too rushed. I'd rather give the mother more time to see if it stretches on its own. Everyone is so rushed these days. They always want to hurry it up. Just don't want to wait and see.'

The main point made by those at the other end of the scale, who said that episiotomies occurred at less than 30 per cent of deliveries, was: 'They're not done routinely here. In some places every primigravida has one which I'm dead against. They're done here if the need arises.'

Views on women's choices and preferences

Most midwives, 72 per cent, thought that the women they were involved with had about the right amount of choice over induction, while a quarter felt they should have more choice.[3] Some of their

---

[3] 'What choice do the women you are involved with have about being induced?' 'Do you feel that women should be given more or less choice about that than they are – or is it about right?'

expectations and standards over this did not seem high, as these comments from some who felt women had the right amount of choice suggest: 'They don't have any – it's a vicious circle. If you gave them all a choice, well, you could have the ones with genuine medical reasons refusing'; 'Not a lot. All women can say no in theory but in practice they aren't allowed to'; 'I've never seen a doctor ask about it . . . I think the sister would explain the choice to some'; 'No choice. The obstetrician will have told her. One refused but she was induced eventually when she came in.'

Other descriptions of what the midwives thought was a reasonable choice were:

> 'It's explained to them. They are told they will be started off after the E D D. If someone feels strongly against it they are not forced to have it done. It is explained to them that it is in the best interests of the baby. If they refuse then we accept it.'

> 'The doctor explains to them the reason why they are being induced and they are always willing to come in and be induced.'

> 'You explain what's going to happen. They trust you as a medical person and they accept facts.'

Some situations where they thought the mother should have more choice were: 'They're usually frightened. No choice, just told about the date. There's no question of them having a say'; 'Very little [choice]. They don't seem to question it somehow. I'm sure I would!'; 'Not a great deal. They are told what's going to happen and I suppose if they object they would say so.'

A fifth of the midwives thought women were not given enough explanation about induction. Some of their comments were: 'It depends who's on duty. Often we walk round at night and ask if they know what's going to happen and they'll say no'; 'I have my doubts. I don't think they're told enough in the clinic. The general theory in the clinic is speed. They're short of time constantly.' Descriptions of what were seen as satisfactory explanations were:

> 'They're told exactly what is going to happen. We're going to rupture membranes artificially and that we stop putting oxytocin in the drip once they're established in labour. Also we explain the labour is going to be slightly different and they might go straight into having contractions instead of maybe backache and slight pain.'

> 'Quite a bit. I usually go and explain the whole procedure. I think

it's important to alleviate their anxieties and then they're all right.'

'The ladies attending parent-craft classes have full explanations about induction during labour talks. With patients who miss parent-craft classes we do try and explain at ante-natal clinic, and when they're admitted the night before induction they have a complete explanation by the midwife.'

'The procedure was explained to them in terms they could abosrb.'

The views of midwives and obstetricians about who usually explains to women who are to be induced what is involved in an induction are compared in *Table 81*. Both groups mentioned more than two types of person on average. The person most commonly mentioned by the midwives was the staff midwife – the one least often reported by the obstetricians. The situation was reversed when the proportions indicating the consultant are considered.

Table 81   Views of obstetricians and midwives about who usually explains to women what is involved in induction

	Obstetricians	Midwives
	%	%
Consultant	83	33
Registrar	68	37
Houseman	43	37
Sister	32	46
Staff midwife	18	49
Other	4	17
Vague	3	3
Number of professionals (= 100%)	378	309*

* Those with no experience of induction were not asked this question and have been omitted.

When the midwives were divided into sisters, staff midwives, and others, 52 per cent of the sisters said the sister usually gave the explanations (39 per cent of other midwives said this), and 60 per cent of staff midwives (compared with 43 per cent of other midwives) said the staff midwives usually did so. In one sense it seems encouraging that each professional group identified themselves as the group most often involved in giving explanations, but when it is recalled that two-fifths of the women who had an induction expressed some dissatisfaction with the information they were given about this, it is clear that there is no room for complacency and some evidence that professionals' perceptions of explanations may be inadequate from the patients' viewpoint.

Midwives, like obstetricians, seemed to overestimate women's preferences for induction. On average they estimated that 40 per cent would prefer to have their babies induced if they were offered this shortly before the baby was due. They also, again like the obstetricians, overestimated women's preferences for epidurals – but not if the estimate of women preferring them is confined to those who had had an epidural. Quite unlike obstetricians, they also overestimated the proportion who would prefer a home birth. The figures are in *Table 82.*

In making their estimates of what proportion of women would prefer various arrangements, they may have attached undue weight to the unusual and the vociferous, since in all instances they over-

Table 82   Midwives' estimates of the proportion of mothers who would prefer various arrangements

	Induction	Epidural	Home birth
	%	%	%
80% or more	7	4	5
70% < 80%	10	5	5
60% < 70%	7	3	5
50% < 60%	19	13	14
40% < 50%	8	9	9
30% < 40%	6	11	7
20% < 30%	12	16	16
10% < 20%	12	14	13
5% < 10%	9	10	13
Less than 5%	10	15	13
Average proportion	40%	32%	33%
Number of midwives (= 100%)	367	345	370
Proportion of all mothers who said they would prefer arrangement	8%	16%	18%
Number of mothers (= 100%)	2174	2166	2175

estimated the demand for a procedure preferred by a minority.

Midwives under forty-five were asked about their personal pre-ferences if they were to have a baby – or another baby if they had already had one. Eleven per cent said they would prefer an induction, 10 per cent would prefer an epidural, and 20 per cent would prefer a home birth. So their replies are similar to the mothers', except that rather fewer of the midwives would opt for an epidural.

Characteristics of the midwives

Over two-fifths of the midwives, 44 per cent, were under thirty-five, 29 per cent were aged thirty-five to forty-four, 18 per cent aged forty-five to fifty-four, and 9 per cent aged fifty-five to sixty-four. None were older. Just over half, 53 per cent, were sisters, over a third, 37 per cent, were staff midwives, and 10 per cent were nursing officers. Nursing officers as a group were older: 51 per cent were forty-five or more compared with 29 per cent of the sisters and 15 per cent of the staff midwives; and, at the other end of the scale, 15 per cent of the staff midwives were under twenty-five, against only 1 per cent of the others.

Over half, 57 per cent, were married, 39 per cent were single and had never been married, leaving 2 per cent who were widowed and 2 per cent divorced or separated. Seventy per cent of the married, or 43 per cent of all the midwives, had children of their own. More of the staff midwives than of the sisters were married and had children; the majority of nursing officers had never married, and even among those who had few of them had any children (see *Table 83*).

A third of the midwives worked part-time, and this proportion was highest, 44 per cent, among the older midwives aged fifty-five or more. It was a quarter for the sisters, half for staff nurses, and only one out of forty for nursing officers. Two-thirds of those with children worked part-time, as did a fifth of those who were married with no children. Only 5 per cent were currently doing any work in the community.[4] Over two-thirds, 69 per cent, had been born in England or Wales, 2 per cent in Scotland, 7 per cent in Ireland, 14 per cent in Africa or the West Indies, 2 per cent in India, Pakistan, or Bangladesh, and the rest elsewhere. English was the native language of 84 per cent; for the rest, the interviewers rated their English as good in all but four cases, 1 per cent of all midwives, whose English was rated as fair.

---

[4] 'Do you work in hospital only or sometimes in the community?'

Table 83 Midwives' rank, marital status, and children

	Staff midwife	*Sister*	*Nursing officer*	*All midwives*
	%	%	%	%
Never married	30	41	60	39
Married, no children	12	21	25	18
Married, some children	58	38	15	43
Number of midwives (= 100%)	140	201	40	385

One in eight of the midwives had been working in the same hospital for less than a year, and a fifth for between one and two years, but one-fifth had been there for between five and ten years, and almost another fifth, 18 per cent, for ten years or more. Length of stay did not seem to be related to the size of the hospital.

Some variations between midwives

To what extent, if at all, did these various characteristics relate to their views of induction and other aspects of obstetric care? More of the older midwives, aged thirty-five or over, than of their younger colleagues thought that the increase in inductions had decreased the job satisfaction of midwives, 35 per cent against 26 per cent. But there was no variation with age in the proportions who thought it had made the experience more or less pleasant for women. Neither did their views on the effect for women vary with their rank or whether they worked full- or part-time. However, more of those who were or had been married than of those who had never been married felt it had made the experience for women less pleasant, 52 per cent compared with 41 per cent. But there was no difference among the married between those who had children and the childless.

A rather similar pattern emerged in relation to their views about the choice that women were given over induction: 17 per cent of the single thought they should have more choice, 31 per cent of those who had ever been married. Again there was no difference between those with and without children among the marrieds, nor between midwives of different rank. Neither did this vary with age. But more of those working part-time than of those working full-time thought women should have more choice: 35 per cent compared with 20 per cent.

So there is some suggestion that married midwives and those working part-time may be more critical and questioning of technical procedures and the lack of involvement of women in decisions about their care.

Hopes for the future

Towards the end of the interview, midwives were asked what they would most like to happen if more resources were available for the maternity services. Many of their suggestions related to buildings, equipment, and staffing.

Comments about buildings reflect the unevenness of services: 'Appalling bathroom and toilet facilities here and no bidets. The ward I work on there are eleven patients with one bathroom and one toilet. We need day-rooms. We could do with a new hospital'; 'A new maternity wing. It's dreadful the running around you do here'; 'Nothing really. Everything seems adequate here at the moment. We have no problems.'

Desired equipment ranged from nappies and wraps to disposable items, incubators, and monitoring equipment, but it was 'more monitoring equipment' that was mentioned most often.

Some wishes for more staff were: 'We could do with a permanent doctor, someone at least on call for twenty-four hours so that you wouldn't have to rush round_____looking for a doctor in a case of fetal distress. It would cut down the rushed cases to_____'; 'Ideally to have enough midwives to give individual care'; 'More nursing and medical staff. You can do without machinery but it's important to mums to have somebody there to hold their hands and tell them how well they are doing. There is nothing worse than going hours on end and nobody there.'

By no means all the wishes were for material things or an increase in numbers of people. Several wanted policy changes and an emphasis on different types of service:

'Smaller hospital units where the patient can have more individual attention. Smaller and more frequent ante-natal clinics so the patient doesn't have to wait so long.'

'A lot more home deliveries, or patients just coming into hospital to deliver the babies and going home straight afterwards. This would lower the depression rate after the birth, especially for women who already have small children at home and worry about them.'

'I'd like to see the nurses more interested in post-natal care and spending more time on helping mothers to breast feed the baby.'

'Family planning services on the maternity unit. A lot of patients once they have gone home do not make an effort to go to see their family planning doctor. The service should be more readily available when they are in hospital.'

'More staff in the field to do more home deliveries.'

'If there were plenty of resources available I would really like to see these young mums having their babies in their own surroundings, in their own homes, although I do realize it's safer to come into hospital. They're much more contented and settled, there is a difference.'

'Mothers going home earlier with *all* the midwives going out to visit. A forty-eight hour stay in hospital and support at home if needed.'

'I'd like less inductions. Hospitals induce too many women, especially when they're at term and they've got a few empty beds, so they're induced for administrative convenience.'

Conclusions

Midwives, as a group, were more sceptical than obstetricians about the advantages of the recent increase in inductions and more inclined to perceive disadvantages. There are two possible explanations of this difference between them.

The first relates to the differing relationship of obstetricians and midwives to mothers and babies. Midwives generally have a closer and more continuous one, and being women they are likely to identify more easily and readily with the experiences and reactions of childbearing women. They will be in a better position to observe many of the effects of induction on mothers' physical and emotional comfort, and they may attach more importance to the reactions of mothers.

Another explanation relates to the relationship between obstetricians and midwives. Induction, and other technological changes, may be seen as shifting the balance of power to greater medical dominance. Midwives may resent this, and prefer more home births and a greater emphasis on 'natural' childbirth because they would be more powerful in those situations.

Probably both explanations contribute to the differing attitudes of midwives and obstetricians to induction, epidural anaesthesia, and home births. The extent to which midwives can be seen as identifying with mothers is limited in the sense that many accepted, apparently uncritically, the doctors' power to make decisions about induction without taking into account mothers' views and preferences.

9 Discussion

In this last chapter I try to bring together the implications of the study and put them into perspective. I start by reviewing the findings on induction policies and practices and go on to look at women's reactions to their experiences of spontaneous and induced labour. After that I consider the implications of these findings for other innovatory and interventionist procedures. This leads to a discussion of ways in which women's preferences could play a greater part in the shaping of maternity services and of other reforms that are needed.

Induction policies and practices

In the introduction, three types of explanation for the rise in inductions were discussed: first, the most straightforward and respectable one that it reduced perinatal mortality and morbidity, cut down the proportion of long labours, and made the experience of labour more pleasant for mothers; second, that it had increased the power and prestige of obstetricians; and, third, that it made the organization and staffing of maternity services easier and more efficient and was more convenient for mothers.

Results from other studies suggest that the rise in inductions had contributed little to the fall in the perinatal mortality rate. Nevertheless, it is clear from our survey of obstetricians that most of them believed it had done so, and this view, although it now appears to be mistaken, was clearly a major contributory factor in the increase.

The claim that the length of labour was reduced by induction was substantiated by our study, but of course this could be achieved by acceleration and does not necessitate intervention before labour starts. The contention that it had made labour more pleasant for women was not borne out. Only a minority, 40 per cent, of obstetricians felt that it had done so, and almost half the midwives, 47 per cent, thought it had made the experience *less* pleasant. The data from the mothers showed an overwhelming rejection of induction as a preferred way of starting labour, but at the same time the majority of those who had had one seemed to adjust to the experience reasonably well: similar proportions of those whose labour started spontaneously and those who had an induction regarded their labour as a pleasurable experience, and a tenth of each group described it as a nightmare. Again contrary to much opinion, induced labours were not rated as more painful by the women, but more of those who were induced were given pain relief. So neither the claims for induction in this respect nor the more extreme claims against it were substantiated.

It is difficult to confirm or rebut the view that induction policy has been influenced by the desire of some obstetricians to increase their power and prestige. Cynics may feel that the falling birth rate is likely to accentuate any such tendency and those who favour such a theory will probably see three of the findings from the study as giving some support to their views. The first is the overall lack of any relationship between induction and any risk factors associated with characteristics of the mothers, while at the same time induction rates varied widely between areas and between hospitals. The second is that relatively few obstetricians with university appointments induced a high proportion of their patients. The third is that both obstetricians and midwives perceived the rise in inductions as increasing rather than decreasing the job satisfaction of obstetricians. However, all these observations may be interpreted in other ways. The variation in induction rates between obstetricians was shown to be related to their views on the effects of induction. Obstetricians with university appointments may be trend leaders and are possibly no less or more influenced than other obstetricians by a desire to increase their power or prestige. Finally, job satisfactions too relate to perceptions of other outcomes of induction.

This last relationship may be attributed in part at any rate to a halo effect. It was probably not difficult for obstetricians who enjoyed the technology and activity of inductions to convince themselves of the advantages of induction in instances where their colleagues whose preference was for less activity and intervention would remind themselves of the hazards of 'meddlesome midwifery' and the rewards of 'masterly inactivity'.

There is no evidence from this study of the widescale use of induction simply for the sake of convenience. If some consultants were adopting such a policy they either changed it, concealed it, or did not respond to our questionnaire. In addition, they convinced their patients and the midwives that the inductions were being done for other, medical, reasons. Finally, their success was limited : they may have cut down the number of births on Sundays and in the early hours of the morning, but half their obstetric colleagues and two-thirds of the midwives did not feel that the increase in induction had made the running of maternity departments easier. However, it was clear from the study that induction was used by substantial proportions of obstetricians in situations where there was not a clear-cut medical indication. 'Expedient' rather than 'convenient' is probably a more appropriate description of the situation in which induction was carried out to ensure that expert staff would be available when the baby was born.

Women's views and experiences of induced and spontaneous labour

So far I have been reviewing the possible explanations for the rise in inductions and seeing how far the study findings supported these explanations. But the main purpose in doing the survey of mothers was to find out about their views and experiences of induced as compared with spontaneous labour. There had been reports of the dehumanizing of childbirth, the mechanistic approach which made childbirth an alienating and warping experience, and of the deleterious physical and emotional effects on the mother, on the baby, and on their relationship. What were the findings of the study in relation to these accusations?

The most clear-cut verdict was that the great majority of women on the survey would not want an induction if they were having another baby. Although a higher proportion of those whose labour was induced this time than of those whose labour started spontaneously would prefer an induction next time, the fact that among those with experience of the procedure over three-quarters would prefer *not* to have an induction contrasts markedly with their preferences for a home or hospital confinement or for having or not having an epidural. For these types of care, between 63 per cent and 91 per cent voted for the same arrangement as last time. And this vote against induction was in response to a question that stressed the positive sides of induction and in spite of the evidence that the majority of women find the latter part of their pregnancy an uncomfortable and frustrating time.

The main reason for the rejection of induction was that it was unnatural. The point that women felt a sense of failure if they did not go into labour spontaneously was stressed more often by obstetricians and midwives than by the women themselves.

When the different aspects of pregnancy, labour, and delivery are considered, the case against induction from the mother's point of view seems less overwhelming. There were no differences between those with spontaneous and induced labours in the average length of time they had bad pains, or in the proportions who had breech deliveries, who were left alone at some stage during their labour, whose husbands were present at the birth, who reported anxieties during labour, or who had Caesarean sections. On the debit side, women who were induced more often complained of being thirsty during labour, they more often had assisted deliveries, more of them had to be stitched, and more of them felt unpleasantly restricted during their labour. There were two credits: women who were induced more often had their husbands with them in the early stages of labour and less often minded that they had been left alone at some stage.

The differences after delivery in the baby's health, in the mother's health, and in our rather superficial indicators of the mother and baby relationship between the two groups (induced and spontaneous start to labour) were both few and small. Rather more induced babies had been in a special care unit or nursery and more of them were said to have had jaundice. One potentially significant finding was that more of the women who had been induced reported nerves or depression since the birth. Again the difference was small and needs verification.

The majority of the observed differences were clearly against induction, and this, together with the preference of the great majority of childbearing women for *not* being induced, the lack of evidence about the circumstances in which the benefits of induction outweigh the disadvantages (Chalmers and Richards 1978), and the costs and potential hazards of the procedure, adds to a clear indictment of the routine use of the procedure after the expected date of delivery.

Implications for other innovatory and interventionist procedures

What lessons can be learned from the induction story? How did it happen that a procedure, which had not been carefully evaluated, which involved considerable costs and hazards, and was disliked by childbearing women, came to be used so widely and accepted uncritically? The explanation I think lies in the explosion in technology during the last twenty years which has presented a bewildering number of choices and opportunities to those concerned with and responsible for childbearing services. The possibilities for investigation and intervention have multiplied in a way that may increase the potential power of the obstetrician to reduce maternal and infant mortality and morbidity. At the same time, the extent to which changing obstetric practices and techniques have contributed to the fall in mortality and morbidity is being questioned along with the value and effect on medical practices more generally (McKeown 1976). It is also increasingly recognized that effective techniques carry risks which may not be immediately apparent. Inevitably it was some time before the hazard of X-rays in early pregnancy increasing the risk of leukemia in childhood was recognized. It was identified and documented by careful and imaginative epidemiological studies (Stewart, Webb, and Hewitt 1958). To study the potential risks of interventions needs an input of scientific, critical, and detached assessment on a considerable scale. The rate of change makes such assessments all the more necessary and, at the same time, more difficult. One problem is that a technique which may have great potential and value once it has been perfected, may be harmful in the initial experimental phase. This poses ethical as well as scientific problems. Another related difficulty is that techniques may become obsolete by the time they have been evaluated, or other techniques may be developed which modify the use and usefulness of the procedure. An illustration of this is an evaluation of continuous fetal heart rate monitoring in high-risk pregnancy which found that 'the presumptive benefits of electronic fetal monitoring for improving fetal outcome were not found in this study' (Haverkamp et al. 1976). This evaluation has been criticized and dismissed as irrelevant by some obstetricians because more elaborate techniques for monitoring by sampling fetal blood have now been developed and were not used in this trial.

So, although it may be shocking to scientists from other disciplines to find that many obstetric techniques and policies (episiotomies, ante-natal care, various types of anaesthesia, home or hospital delivery, induction, acceleration) have not been appropriately evaluated, a simple demand for randomized control trials is not enough. A sceptic might feel that even if all current interventions were shown to be ineffective or harmful, the time taken to demonstrate this and the rate at which techniques are developing would mean that by the time the results were available they would be liable to be dismissed as irrelevant since newer or modified methods would have superseded the ones that had been evaluated. And, while an optimist would feel that such a demonstration would have a salutory and beneficial effect on the thinking and behaviour of practitioners, he should take into account the probable optimism of those practitioners about their latest discovery and their proclivity to action and intervention (Friedson 1970).

Randomized control trials have other disadvantages besides the time they take. To withhold an established technique may be viewed as unethical even if the technique has not been evaluated. Even techniques that are recognized as experimental are likely to have their advocates and critics. Chalmers and Richards (1978) argue persuasively that 'medical ethics demand that if patients are to be involved in experimentation then it should be controlled rather than uncontrolled'. But many procedures cannot be applied in a 'double blind' way and the effect of the doctor on the outcome cannot be ignored. To ask a practitioner to perform a procedure he regards as unnecessary or to withhold one when he thinks it is appropriate is likely to have a negative effect. In some situations it may be more appropriate to identify and then compare units with different practices, in the same way as Chalmers, Lawson, and Turnbull (1976) compared the two units with different practices on induction in Cardiff.

The present study has shown that there are considerable variations in the policies and techniques that predominate in different areas and different hospitals: in some hospitals particular techniques may be used almost routinely, in others hardly at all. With this approach of exploiting the existing differences and using them as a natural experiment, it is of course necessary to ascertain that the units are covering similar populations, or to control or exclude those with certain characteristics so that the two groups are comparable.

A major difficulty in both randomized control trials and 'natural experiments' is taking into account all the relevant effects of the intervention. A procedure may have a desired outcome and the extent to which the outcome is achieved will be assessed in the evaluation. Any reasonable evaluation will also take into account the side effects of the procedure, its long-term effects, and its costs in money, manpower, and resources. In the past the social and psychological effects have rarely been considered. Now, although increasing attention is paid to the comfort and to the social and emotional needs of childbearing women, this study has shown that there is still a long way to go.

Women's voices

'A mother should have learned about induction at ante-natal classes and if later it appears that induction would be the safer course of action for her, she should have every opportunity of discussing it with professional advisers. Knowing what is likely to be involved, she can make a fully informed decision about it.'

This is the view of the Department of Health and Social Security expounded in the discussion paper *Reducing the Risk* (1977). On these criteria, over three-fifths of the women in the study had *not* discussed induction with a professional during their pregnancy, two-fifths of those who were induced did not feel they were given enough information about it, and two-thirds did not feel they had a choice about it. Among the induced the proportion fulfilling the Department's three criteria was only 15 per cent.

There is clear evidence from the study that many women were not given information they would have liked about various aspects of childbearing. It is also apparent that the large majority, four-fifths, wanted to be involved in making decisions about their care. In the meantime, for the most part they accept, adapt to, and make the best of the information, the choices, and the conditions that are available. They appreciate it when their husbands are 'allowed' to be with them during labour, they think it is wonderful when they are 'given' their babies to hold immediately after the birth, and they are happier when they can feed their babies on demand rather than at fixed times. But when these things do not happen few protest. The more common reaction is to try to view the situation from the other point of view, to explain the authoritarianism in terms of inadequate facilities, staff shortages, and other jobs and needs to be met. This prevents them from harbouring grievances and enables them to maintain a good relationship with the people and the organization whose power they are in.

The women's movement may have raised expectations and heightened awareness among some women, but it has a long way to go in giving women confidence and ability to challenge and change services rather than passively to accept them.

The women's movement

What part can the women's movement play in seeing that childbearing services take account of the social, psychological, and physical needs of women and babies? In the USA the movement has been highly critical of many current obstetric practices but, as Macintyre (1977) has pointed out, it has created a myth of a golden age of childbirth in earlier times or primitive societies which is quite unrealistic. Such myths can lead to movements for 'do-it-yourself obstetrics' in unsuitable conditions. In addition, such myths are likely to alienate obstetricians and midwives since, by implication, they deride their profession and achievements. The pendulum seems to have swung from accepting services to rejecting them; from idolizing doctors to vilifying them. I would like to see more emphasis on co-operation and more energies directed towards changing services. I suggest three ways of stimulating appropriate changes.

First, women should ask questions. We should encourage each other and steel ourselves to ask and we should rid ourselves of the habit of waiting and hoping that we will be told the things we want to know. We must learn to think quickly of appropriate follow-up questions so that we are not fobbed off with a reply which on reflection we realize did not answer our question. We may feel reluctant to expose our ignorance but we should try to overcome this feeling, and if doctors or nurses ever try to ridicule us for asking or for not knowing we should unite in condemning such a despicable reaction.

Second, we must make our wishes and preferences known. It is no good just hoping that certain things will happen. If we care about them we should make this clear and if our stated preferences are ignored we should ask why.

Third, we should insist on being involved in important decisions. This is probably the most difficult task. Faced by a demand that a woman should be able to choose whether or not to have a particular procedure performed, some doctors are apt to resort to what has been nicely described as 'shroud waving'. We need to know the relative risks and to recognize that all courses of action involve some risk. We should all rebel against the paternalism of the doctor who refuses explanation and simply insists that he knows best.

If women had asked more questions, made their preferences and dislikes more widely known, and had insisted on taking part in the decisions about whether to be induced or not, I doubt if anything like so many inductions would have been carried out.

Other reforms

But the pressures for change and improvement should come not only from childbearing women. This study has highlighted the need for a more scientific, questioning, and self-critical attitude among many obstetricians, particularly in relation to the possible new techniques that confront them. In addition, authoritarianism and paternalism need to give way to a greater willingness to inform and discuss. Midwives have a vital part to play in the development of a childbearing service in which mothers play a more dominant and less subservient role. They can facilitate and participate in the flow of information, ensure that mothers' needs and preferences are communicated and not ignored or suppressed, and encourage questioning.

Another basic issue which needs to be tackled is inequality. It is abundantly clear from this study that the wives and children of men in unskilled jobs were at a disadvantage in many respects. Their babies were lighter and fewer were breast fed. The wives were less often sure of their dates, they went to ante-natal classes later, fewer of them went to preparation classes, they were less likely to be admitted to hospital during pregnancy, fewer had their husbands with them at the birth, and fewer had a post-natal examination. None of these differences are surprising, and many have been found in other studies. Several relate to the use of preventive services which women in social class V may view as irrelevant or find alienating or unacceptable (McKinlay and Dutton 1974).

What has been less well documented is the extent to which they are deprived of information and of opportunities for discussion with professional people. This was associated with a desire for more information about a wide range of topics related to childbearing. It would appear that some doctors and nurses feel that women in the lower social classes do not want or need information and choices as much as middle-class women. In practice they often need more information because of their earlier deprivation and, although a higher proportion of women in social class V than in social class I said they did not want to be involved in the decision-making process, the great majority, four-fifths, of both groups did. Recognition of these needs is long overdue.

So too is recognition of the needs of those women who have had a still birth for personal information and support. Understanding what happened will often be a helpful preliminary to accepting and coming to terms with it. But as such tragedies become more infrequent it seems that hospital doctors, midwives, general practitioners, and health visitors may feel less able to cope with them and may be reluctant to offer sympathy and understanding. All too often women find they are ignored or avoided when they most need someone who is willing to listen and respond to their anxieties and their grief.

Women, partly because of the women's movement, are increasingly conscious of the indignities of labour. Dignity can only be achieved through a true partnership between parents and professionals.

Appendix I
The sample of areas and births

The sample design was a two-stage one, the first stage units being twenty-four registration districts, or combinations of registration districts, selected with probability proportional to the number of births occurring in the area. Then in each chosen area the Office of Population Censuses and Surveys selected a random sample of 100 legitimate live births: fifty from births registered in July 1975 and fifty in August 1975. This combination of selecting equal numbers of births from each study area while areas were chosen with probability proportional to their number of births means that each birth registered in England and Wales during the study period had an equal chance of being included in the sample. Further details of the way the areas were chosen are given next.

The way the areas were chosen

To select the twenty-four registration districts, the total number of live births registered in England and Wales during the period April to November 1974 were summed for each county and conurbation.

It was necessary to take the births occurring in the area rather than the births to women normally resident in the area because we wanted to approach mothers within the four months after the birth. Data about births to women normally resident in an area would not have been available so soon. The period April to November 1974 was chosen because these were the most recent data available at the time we needed to select our sample of areas. (We wanted to identify the areas for the main inquiry before selecting areas for the pilot study.)

The counties and conurbations were then listed in geographical order from North to South and the number of births summed cumulatively. (The figures for this were taken from the Registrar General's Weekly Returns.) The total number of births (431,307) was divided by twenty-four to give the sampling interval (17,971) and a number under this selected from a book of random

Table A Study areas

Registration District(s)	Areas covered	County
Central Cleveland	Middlesbrough, Stockton-on-Tees, Langbaurgh*	Cleveland
Newcastle-upon-Tyne	Newcastle-upon-Tyne	Tyne and Wear
Ryedale/Whitby/Scarborough	Helmsley, Malton, Pickering, Whitby, Scarborough	North Yorkshire
Halifax/Todmorden	Brighouse, Halifax, Sowerby Bridge, Todmorden	West Yorkshire
Macclesfield/Vale Royal/Halton	Knutsford, Macclesfield, Northwich, Winsford, Runcorn, Widnes	Cheshire
Barton/Trafford/Leigh	Eccles, Swinton, Trafford, Leigh	Greater Manchester
Preston and South Ribble/Ribble Valley/West Lancashire	Leyland, Preston and South Ribble, Ribble Valley,* Tarleton, West Lancashire	Lancashire
Ashbourne/Belper/Ilkeston	Ashbourne, Belper, Ripley, Ilkeston, Long Eaton, Wirksworth	Derbyshire
Brackley/Daventry/Northampton/Towcester	Brackley, Daventry, Northampton, Towcester	Northamptonshire
Bridgnorth/Clun/Ludlow/Wrekin	Bridgnorth, Cleobury Mortimer, Wenlock, Bishop's Castle and Clun, Craven Arms, Ludlow, Dawley, Newport, Oakengates, Shifnal, Wellington	Salop
Birmingham	Birmingham	West Midlands
Meriden	Meriden, Marston Green	West Midlands

(continued)

Registration District(s)	Areas covered	County
Norwich/Norwich Outer/Depwade/East Dereham/Wayland	Norwich, Norwich Outer, Diss, East Dereham, Thetford	Norfolk
Slough/Windsor and Maidenhead	Slough, Maidenhead, Windsor	Berkshire
Southend-on-Sea	Southend-on-Sea	Essex
Greenwich	Greenwich	Greater London
Hampstead/St. Pancras	Hampstead, St. Pancras	Greater London
Hillingdon	Hayes, Hillingdon, Ruislip, Uxbridge	Greater London
New Forest/Ringwood & Fordingbridge/Romsey/Southampton	Lymington, New Forest, Ringwood and Fordingbridge, Romsey, Eastleigh, Southampton	Hampshire
Ashford/Dover/Shepway	Ashford, Tenterden, Deal, Dover, Folkestone, Hythe and Romney Marsh	Kent
Surrey Mid-Eastern	Dorking, Epsom and Leatherhead, Epsom Woodcote	Surrey
Bath/Sodbury	Bath, Norton Radstock, Sodbury	Avon
Forest of Dean/Stroud/Gloucester	Forest of Dean, Stroud, Gloucester	Gloucestershire
Blaenaw Gwent/Pontypool	Abertillery, Ebbw Vale and Tredegar, Abergavenny, Pontypool	Gwent

* Part of area.

numbers to give a random starting point (1,419). The counties or conurbations in which 1,419, 19,390 (1,419 + 17,971), 37,361, etc., fell were then
identified, and within these chosen counties and conurbations a detailed
breakdown of births in the given period for each of the registration districts was
obtained from the Office of Population Censuses and Surveys. When
necessary, the registration districts were grouped together geographically so
that each district or combination of districts had at least 1,000 births registered
during the eight-month period. The numbers of births in these areas were then
listed in the order in which they appeared in *The Official List for 1974* (Office of
Population Censuses and Surveys 1974), summed cumulatively, and the areas
containing the sampling points identified.

The study areas

The areas selected in this way are shown in *Table A*.
   Eight of the twenty-four study areas were in conurbations, three in Greater
London, two in the West Midlands, one in West Yorkshire, one in Greater
Manchester, and one in Tyne and Wear. (In 1974, 14 per cent of the legitimate
live births were in Greater London, and 24 per cent in Metropolitan
Counties.) The stratification from North to South ensured that areas were also
appropriately distributed in this respect. So the sample of areas seems to be
reasonable. What about the resulting sample of births?

The representativeness of the sample of births

As explained in the main body of the report, in each area fifty legitimate births
registered during July 1975 and fifty during August were selected at random
by the Office of Population Censuses and Surveys (OPCS). Multiple births
were treated as a single event since basically we wanted a sample of mothers.
Out of this sample of 2,400 mothers, 91 per cent were successfully interviewed.
Table B   Parity comparisons with OPCS data

OPCS data			*Survey data*
Number of previous live born children	*June quarter*	*September quarter*	*Number of previous pregnancies ending in a live or still birth*
	%	%	%	
0	41.1	43.1	37.5	0
1	39.3	37.3	39.5	1
2	12.8	12.7	15.0	2
3	4.2	4.2	5.8	3
4+	2.6	2.7	2.2	4+
Number of births (= 100%)	135,900	131,900	2,179	

Most of the interviews, 95 per cent, were completed within the five months after the birth.

The question here is, how far is this sample a representative one? Four characteristics can be compared with national data: the number of infant deaths, the place of birth, the mother's parity, and the mother's age.

Twenty-five of the live born babies had died by the time of interview, that is 11.5 per 1,000. In 1975 the neonatality rate (deaths of infants under four weeks of age) was 10.7 per 1,000 live births, and the infant mortality rate (deaths of infants under one year of age) was 15.7, so our rate, based on deaths in the first four or five months, is probably slightly low but of the right order.

In 1974, 4.4 per cent of births in England took place at home, and the proportion in our sample of legitimate births in England and Wales in July and August 1975 was precisely the same.

Turning to parity, in the sample there seemed to be an under-representation of mothers who had had no previous pregnancies ending in a live or still birth. Comparisons with Office of Population Censuses and Surveys data relate to the number of previous live born children to women married once only. The figures are in *Table B*.

The differences are statistically significant, but they probably arise because of different definitions and populations. Two of these differences would tend to a reduction in nulliparous women in the sample. One is the exclusion from the OPCS data of women married more than once. The other is that OPCS data relate to previous live born children, whereas the definition of parity on this survey was pregnancies ending in a live or still birth. The other difference is that multiple births were only counted as a single pregnancy on the survey, whereas the OPCS data relate to previous live born children. This may account for some of the difference at the other end of the distribution.

The age distribution of the mothers in our sample is shown in *Table C* and compared with Office of Population Censuses and Surveys data for all mothers of legitimate live births in England and Wales in 1975. The small proportion of older mothers, aged forty or more, is under-represented in our sample. Possibly they were less willing to be interviewed.

Table C Mother's age: comparisons with OPCS data

Mother's age	OPCS data	Survey data
	%	%
Under 20	7.8	6.7
20–24	31.6	31.9
25–29	39.4	41.3
30–34	15.3	15.2
35–39	4.7	4.4
40+	1.2	0.5
Total (= 100%)	548,554	2,178

Appendix II
Statistical significance and sampling errors

There are a number of factors, particularly the nature of the data and the stage at which precise hypotheses were often formulated, that violate some of the conditions in which statistical tests of significance apply and make interpretation difficult. For this reason they are rarely referred to in the text, in an attempt to avoid the appearance of spurious precision which the presentation of such tests might seem to imply. But, in the absence of more satisfactory techniques, these tests have been used to give some indication of the probability of differences occurring by chance.

Chi-square, t, chi-square trend tests, and tests for differences between proportions have been applied constantly when looking at the data from this survey, and have influenced decisions about what differences to present and how much verbal 'weight' to attach to them. In general, attention has not been drawn to any difference that statistical tests suggest might have occurred by chance five or more times in 100.

Another difficulty about presenting results from a study like this, with over 300 items of basic information from the mothers alone, is that of selection. Inevitably not all cross-analyses are carried out – only about 2,000 – and only a fraction of these are presented, which of course gives rise to difficulty in interpreting significance. Positive results are more often shown than negative ones. Readers may sometimes wonder why certain further analyses are not reported. Often, but not always, the analysis will have been done but the result found to be negative or inconclusive.

Table D shows the sampling error for a number of characteristics. (For the appropriate formula see Gray and Corlett (1950).) Because of the wide variations between areas the design effect is greater than two for the proportion of home births, of those having an epidural, and of those whose husbands were present at some stage during labour.

Table D Sampling errors

	Value in total sample	Range in 24 study areas	Sampling error	Estimated random sampling error*	Range ± two sampling errors	Design effect**
Proportion of induced births	23.9%	6%–39%	1.6%	0.9%	20.7%–27.1%	1.8
Proportion of home births	4.4%	0%–17%	1.0%	0.4%	2.4%–6.4%	2.5
Proportion given an epidural	5.1%	0%–22%	1.4%	0.5%	2.3%–7.9%	2.8
Proportion having their first child	37.5%	27%–44%	0.9%	1.0%	35.7%–39.3%	0.9
Proportion in social classes IV and V	20.5%	9%–35%	1.1%	0.9%	18.3%–22.7%	1.2
Proportion reporting fathers present at some stage during labour	68.9%	50%–89%	2.4%	1.0%	64.1%–73.7%	2.4
Proportion preferring an induction next time	7.8%	2%–13%	0.6%	0.6%	6.6%–9.0%	1.0

* If a random sample throughout the country, that is, $\sqrt{\dfrac{p.q}{n}}$.

** The ratio of the sampling error with the given two-stage sample design to the estimated random sampling error.

173

Appendix III
Classification of social class

As our index of social class, we took the father's occupation and classified it according to the Registrar General's *Classifications of Occupations* (Office of Population Censuses and Surveys 1970). This distinguishes six 'social class' groups:

I   Professional, etc., occupations
II   Intermediate occupations
III Skilled occupations
    (N) Non-manual
    (M) Manual
IV   Partly skilled occupations
V   Unskilled occupations.

These classes are intended to reflect 'the general standing within the community of the occupations concerned'. In a number of instances the main differences that emerge are between what can be described as the 'middle class' and 'working class', the former being most of the non-manual occupations – the Registrar General's social classes I, II, and III non-manual – and the latter almost entirely manual – III manual, IV, and V.

Data about this were obtained from two sources, the birth certificates and the interviews. They were both coded, independently, at the Institute for Social Studies in Medical Care. The distributions are compared in *Table E*.

As in an earlier study (Cartwright 1976), a relatively small proportion of occupations recorded at the interviews were classified as unskilled, 4 per cent, compared with 6 per cent of those on the birth certificates. Apart from this small difference the distributions were almost identical.

A cross-analysis of data from the birth certificates and the interviews showed that 80 per cent were in precisely the same category, 11 per cent differed by one category, and 9 per cent by more than one. The information from the birth certificates and the interviews related to different points in time, and there may

Table E   Social class distributions based on data from birth certificates and from interviews

	Birth certificates	Interviews
	%	%
I Professional	9	9
II Intermediate	18	19
III Skilled{Non-manual	11	11
III Skilled{Manual	41	42
IV Partly skilled	15	15
V Unskilled	6	4
Number classified (= 100%)	2088	2109
Proportion not classified	4%	3%

have been some genuine changes in the four- to five-month period.

Data from the birth certificates have generally been used in the report as these were available even when the mothers were not interviewed. This was also done in *Parents and Family Planning Services* (Cartwright 1970) and *How Many Children?* (Cartwright 1976).

Appendix IV
Classification of cause of
still birth

The cause of still birth was classified from data on the still-birth certificate in two different ways. The first related to the main cause and should be comparable to information classified and published by the Office of Population Censuses and Surveys. The second relates to all contributory factors mentioned on the certificate. Slightly different groupings were used for the two classifications which are shown in *Table F* alongside data for all still births in England and Wales in 1975.

A comparison of national data for England and Wales with the survey data shows a rather higher proportion of the survey still births being classified as due to ill-defined causes (anoxia, hypoxia, immaturity, maceration, or unknown causes) and a somewhat lower proportion as due to conditions of the placenta (other than placenta praevia or premature separation).

When all causes are considered it is shown that immaturity was a contributory factor in 9 per cent of the survey still births, congenital abnormalies in 27 per cent, and anoxic or hypoxic conditions in 26 per cent.

In the main body of the report the proportion induced has been considered in relation to the main cause only. When all causes are taken into account, 54 per cent of those for whom toxaemia was recorded were induced. At the other end of the scale, two of the eighteen, 11 per cent, for which immaturity was mentioned as a contributory factor were induced: for one of these toxaemia was the main cause while for the other it was placental insufficiency.

Table F   Cause of still birth

Cause (and ICD number*)	England and Wales 1975**	Survey data Main cause	Survey data All causes
	%	%	%
Maternal conditions unrelated to pregnancy (760–61)	4	2	5
Toxaemias of pregnancy (762)	9	12	13
Difficult labour (764–68)	3	3	14
Other complications of pregnancy/childbirth (769)	6	6	
Placenta praevia, premature separation of placenta (770.0, 770.1)	10	10	31
Other conditions of placenta (770.2–770.9)	17	11	
Conditions of umbilical cord (771)	8	9	11
Congenital abnormalities of the nervous system (740–43)	19	19	27
Other and unspecified congenital abnormalities (744–59)	4	4	
Anoxia and hypoxic conditions N.E.S.*** (776)	6		26
Immaturity (777)	1		9
Maceration (779.00)	4	16 → 22	8
Unknown (779.9)	5		6
Haemolytic disease of newborn (774–75)	2	1	4
Other conditions	2	1	
Number of still births (= 100%)	6295	196	

* International Classification of Diseases 1976.
** Office of Population Censuses and Survey (1977) *Mortality Statistics Childhood.*
*** N.E.S. Not elsewhere specified.

References

ANDERSON, A. B. M., TURNBULL, A. C., and BAIRD, D. (1968) The influence of induction of labour on Caesarean section rate, duration of labour and perinatal mortality in Aberdeen primigravidae between 1938 and 1966. *Journal of Obstetrics and Gynaecology of the British Commonwealth* **75**: 800–11.

BAIRD, D. (1960) The evolution of modern obstetrics. *Lancet* **2**: 557–64, 609–14.

BAIRD, D. and THOMSON, A. M. (1969) Reduction of perinatal mortality by improving standards of obstetric care. In, N. R. Butler and E. D. Alberman (eds) *Perinatal Problems*. Edinburgh and London: E. and S. Livingstone.

BEARD, R., BRUDENELL, M., DUNN, P., and FAIRWEATHER, D. (eds) (1976) *The Management of Labour*. London: The Royal College of Obstetricians and Gynaecologists.

BRITISH MEDICAL JOURNAL (1976) A policy of despair. *British Medical Journal* **1**: 787–88.

BOURNE, S. (1968) The psychological effects of still births on women and their doctors. *Journal of the Royal College of General Practitioners* **16**: 103–12.

BROWN, G. W., BHROLCHAIN, M., and HARRIS, T. (1975) Social class and psychiatric disturbance among women in an urban population. *Sociology* **9**: 225–54.

BUCHAN, I. C. and RICHARDSON, I. M. (1973) Time study of consultations in general practice. *Scottish Health Studies* No. 27. Edinburgh: Scottish Home and Health Department.

CARTWRIGHT, A. (1970) *Parents and Family Planning Services*. London: Routledge and Kegan Paul.

——(1976) *How Many Children?* London: Routledge and Kegan Paul.

CARTWRIGHT, A. and O'BRIEN, M. (1976) Social class variations in health care and in the nature of general practitioner consultations. *Sociological Review Monograph* **22**: 77–98.

180 References

CARTWRIGHT, A. and SMITH, C. (in press) Some comparisons of data from medical records and from interviews with women who have recently had a live or still birth. *Journal of Biosocial Science.*

CHALMERS, I., LAWSON, J. G., and TURNBULL, A. C. (1976) Evaluation of different approaches to obstetric care: Part I. *British Journal of Obstetrics and Gynaecology* **83**: 921–29.

CHALMERS, I., NEWCOMBE, R. G., and CAMPBELL, H. (1977) Induction of labour and perinatal mortality. *British Medical Journal* **1**: 707–8.

CHALMERS, I. and RICHARDS, M. (1978) Intervention and causal inference in obstetric practice. In, T. Chard and M. Richards (eds) *Benefits and Hazards of the New Obstetrics.* London: Spastics International Medical Publications.

CHALMERS, I., ZLOSNIK, J. E., JOHNS, K. A., and CAMPBELL, H. (1976) Obstetric practice and outcome of pregnancy in Cardiff residents 1965–73. *British Medical Journal* **1**: 735–38.

CHAMBERLAIN, R. *et al.* (1975) *British Births 1970* (Vol. 1) London: Heinemann Medical Books.

COLE, R. A., HOWIE, P. W., and MACNAUGHTON, M. C. (1975) Elective induction of labour—A randomised prospective trial. *Lancet* **1**: 767–72.

DEPARTMENT OF HEALTH AND SOCIAL SECURITY (1976) *On the State of the Public Health for the Year 1975.* London: HMSO.

——(1977a) *Health and Personal Social Services Statistics for England 1976.* London: HMSO.

——(1977b) *On the State of the Public Health for the Year 1976.* London: HMSO.

——(1977c) *Prevention and Health: Reducing the Risk.* London: HMSO.

DUNN, P. M. (1976) Obstetric delivery today: For better or for worse? *Lancet* **1**: 790–93.

EARTHROWL, B. and STACEY, M. (1977) Social class and children in hospital. *Social Science and Medicine* **2**: 83–8.

FEDRICK, J. and YUDKIN, P. (1976) Obstetric practice in the Oxford Record Linkage Study Area from 1965–72. *British Medical Journal* **1**: 738–40.

FREIDSON, E. (1970) *Profession of Medicine.* New York: Dodd, Mead and Co.

GILLIE, L. and GILLIE, O. (1974) The Childbirth Revolution. And, The Vital First Hours. *The Sunday Times*, 13 and 20 October.

GRAY, P. G. and CORLETT, T. (1950) Sampling for the Social Survey. *Journal of the Royal Statistical Society*, Series A (General) **CXIII** (II).

HAVERKAMP, A. D., THOMPSON, H. E., MCFEE, J. G., and CURTIS, C. (1976) The evaluation of continuous fetal heart rate monitoring in high-risk pregnancy. *American Journal of Obstetrics and Gynaecology* **125**: 310–20.

Hospitals and Health Services Year Book 1975, The. London: The Institute of Health Service Administrators.

KITZINGER, S. (1975) Some mothers' experiences of induced labour. Submission to the Department of Health and Social Services from the National Childbirth Trust.

Lancet (1977) The abhorrence of stillbirth. *Lancet* **1**: 1188–90.

LEESON, J. and SMITH, A. (1977) Induction of labour and perinatal mortality. *British Medical Journal* **1**:707.

LEWIS, B. V., RANA, S., and CROOK, E. (1975) Patient response to induction of labour. *Lancet* **1**:1197.

References 181

MACINTYRE, S. (1977) Childbirth: the myth of the Golden Age. *World Medicine* **12** (18): 17–22.

MCKEOWN, T. (1976) *The Role of Medicine: Dream, Mirage or Nemesis?* London: Nuffield Provincial Hospitals Trust.

MCKINLAY, J. B. and DUTTON, D. B. (1974) Social-psychological factors affecting health service utilization. In, S. J. Mushkin (ed.) *Consumer Incentives for Health Care.* New York: Prodist.

MCNAY, M. B., MCILWAINE, G. M., HOWIE, P. W., and MACNAUGHTON, M. C. (1977) Perinatal deaths: analysis by clinical cause to assess value of induction of labour. *British Medical Journal* **1**: 347–50.

MAHLER, H. (1975) Health—a demystification of medical technology. *Lancet* **2**: 829–33.

MARTIN, J. (1978) *Infant Feeding 1975: Attitudes and Practice in England and Wales.* London: HMSO.

O'BRIEN, M. (1978) Home and hospital. *Journal of the Royal College of General Practitioners* **28**: 460–66.

O'DRISCOLL, K., CARROLL, C. J., and COUGHLAN, M. (1975) Selective induction of labour. *British Medical Journal* **4**: 727–29.

OFFICE OF POPULATION CENSUSES AND SURVEYS (1970) *Classification of Occupations 1970.* London: HMSO.

——(1974) *The Official List for 1974* (Part I: List of Registration Offices, etc.) London: OPCS.

——(1977) *Mortality Statistics Childhood.* London: HMSO.

RICHARDS, M. P. M. (1975) Innovation in medical practice: Obstetricians and the induction of labour in Britain. *Social Science & Medicine* **9**: 595–602.

ROBINSON, J. (1974) Having a baby in Britain today – Battery hen mothers and conveyor belt babies. *Doctor*, 18 July.

STEWART, A., WEBB, J., and HEWITT, D. (1958) A survey of childhood malignancies. *British Medical Journal* **1**: 1495–1508.

TIPTON, R. H. and LEWIS, B. V. (1975) Induction of labour and perinatal mortality. *British Medical Journal* **1**: 391.

WALKER, P. A., MARTIN, R. H., and HIGGINBOTTOM, J. (1972) Towards easier childbirth. *Lancet* **2**: 374.

Index

Harris, T., 87
Haverkamp, A. D., 161
health visitors, 90–1
help at home, 82–4
Hewitt, D., 161
Higginbottom, J., 3
home births, 18, 40, 137, 155–6
hormones, 144
hospital, length of stay in, 41–2;
  variations between, 17–19, 56, 162
Hospitals In-Patient Inquiry, 16–17, 30,
  145
Howie, P. W., 4, 30
husbands, 83–4, 86, 163;
  discussions with, 95;
  during labour, 64–8;
  still births and, 37–8, 43
hypoxia, 142

induction, choice by mother, 125;
  definition of, 10–11;
  discussion of, 98–9, 105–6;
  methods of, 10–16;
  midwives' experiences of, 145–7;
  mothers' views on, 103–8;
  non-induction and, 52–70, 91–2,
    114–15;
  numbers of, 16–17;
  policies regarding, 120–6, 157–9;
  reasons for, 25–8;
  reasons for increase in, 1–3;
  voluntary, 53, 103–4, 107, 124
information, about induction, 99–103,
  163;
  about still births, 46–50

Jarman, B., 91
jaundice, 76, 142, 144, 160

Kitzinger, S., 5

labour, 37–9, 52–4, 61–4, 70, 108–12
Lawson, J. G., 5, 17, 162
Leeson, J., 4
Lewis, B. V., 1, 5

machinery, 100, 120–1, 134–5, 140, 141,
  154
Macintyre, S., 164
McKeown, T., 161
McKinlay, J. B., 165
Macnaughton, M. C., 4, 30
McNay, M. B., 4, 20

Mahler, H., 2
Martin, J., 3, 16, 92
membrane sweeps, 10, 12
midwives, 45, 82, 130, 165;
  during labour, 61–4;
  in this study, 8, 152–4;
  still births and, 37, 45, 50;
  views of, 138–56
mothers, age of, 19–20;
  attitudes of, 93–115;
  choices and views of, 159–60, 163–4;
  relationship with baby, 71–92, 142–4;
  selection of for this study, 6, 8

National Childbirth Trust, 5
Newcombe, R. G., 4

O'Brien, M., 52, 92, 112
obstetricians, 3, 16–17;
  comparisons with midwives, 146–8,
    155–6;
  midwives' views on, 14–41;
  NHS and university, 132–5;
  selection of for this study, 6–8;
  views of, 116–37
O'Driscoll, K., 4
Oxford, 3–4
oxytocin, 3, 10, 14, 16, 117, 125, 126, 149

pain, 54–61, 69–70;
  discussions about, 97
parity of mothers, 19–20
perinatal mortality, 1–4, 117, 123, 125,
  157
Perinatal Mortality Survey, 3
pethidine, 55
pitocin, 12
pregnancy, length of, 35, 122, 125
prolapse, 144, 148
prostaglandins, 10, 126

Rana, S., 5
Reducing the Risk, 163
relatives, 42–6, 83, 95
Richards, M., 2, 160, 162
Richardson, I. M., 112
Robinson, J., 3, 5

sleep pattern, babies', 75
Smith, A., 4
social class, 21–4, 66, 83–5, 165–6;
  choice and, 112–15;
  classification of, 174–5;

184 Index